This report contains the collective views of an international group of experts and does not necessarily represent the decisions or the stated policy of the World Health Organization, the International Labour Organization or the United Nations Environment Programme.

Harmonization Project Document No. 6

PART 1: GUIDANCE DOCUMENT ON CHARACTERIZING AND COMMUNICATING UNCERTAINTY IN EXPOSURE ASSESSMENT

PART 2: HALLMARKS OF DATA QUALITY IN CHEMICAL EXPOSURE ASSESSMENT

This project was conducted within the IPCS project on the Harmonization of Approaches to the Assessment of Risk from Exposure to Chemicals.

Published under the joint sponsorship of the World Health Organization, the International Labour Organization and the United Nations Environment Programme, and produced within the framework of the Inter-Organization Programme for the Sound Management of Chemicals.

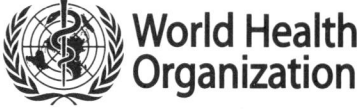

The **International Programme on Chemical Safety (IPCS)**, established in 1980, is a joint venture of the United Nations Environment Programme (UNEP), the International Labour Organization (ILO) and the World Health Organization (WHO). The overall objectives of the IPCS are to establish the scientific basis for assessment of the risk to human health and the environment from exposure to chemicals, through international peer review processes, as a prerequisite for the promotion of chemical safety, and to provide technical assistance in strengthening national capacities for the sound management of chemicals.

The **Inter-Organization Programme for the Sound Management of Chemicals (IOMC)** was established in 1995 by UNEP, ILO, the Food and Agriculture Organization of the United Nations, WHO, the United Nations Industrial Development Organization, the United Nations Institute for Training and Research and the Organisation for Economic Co-operation and Development (Participating Organizations), following recommendations made by the 1992 UN Conference on Environment and Development to strengthen cooperation and increase coordination in the field of chemical safety. The purpose of the IOMC is to promote coordination of the policies and activities pursued by the Participating Organizations, jointly or separately, to achieve the sound management of chemicals in relation to human health and the environment.

WHO Library Cataloguing-in-Publication Data

Uncertainty and data quality in exposure assessment.

(IPCS harmonization project document ; no. 6)

Contents: Part 1: guidance document on characterizing and communicating uncertainty in exposure assessment. Part 2: hallmarks of data quality in chemical exposure assessment.

1.Environmental exposure. 2.Risk assessment - standards. 3.Uncertainty. 4.Data collection - standards. I.International Programme on Chemical Safety. II.Series.

ISBN 978 92 4 156376 5   (NLM classification: QT 140)

© **World Health Organization 2008**

All rights reserved. Publications of the World Health Organization can be obtained from WHO Press, World Health Organization, 20 Avenue Appia, 1211 Geneva 27, Switzerland (tel.: +41 22 791 2476; fax: +41 22 791 4857; e-mail: bookorders@who.int). Requests for permission to reproduce or translate WHO publications — whether for sale or for non-commercial distribution — should be addressed to WHO Press, at the above address (fax: +41 22 791 4806; e-mail: permissions@who.int).

The designations employed and the presentation of the material in this publication do not imply the expression of any opinion whatsoever on the part of the World Health Organization concerning the legal status of any country, territory, city or area or of its authorities, or concerning the delimitation of its frontiers or boundaries. Dotted lines on maps represent approximate border lines for which there may not yet be full agreement.

The mention of specific companies or of certain manufacturers' products does not imply that they are endorsed or recommended by the World Health Organization in preference to others of a similar nature that are not mentioned. Errors and omissions excepted, the names of proprietary products are distinguished by initial capital letters.

All reasonable precautions have been taken by the World Health Organization to verify the information contained in this publication. However, the published material is being distributed without warranty of any kind, either express or implied. The responsibility for the interpretation and use of the material lies with the reader. In no event shall the World Health Organization be liable for damages arising from its use.

Harmonization Project Document No. 6

TABLE OF CONTENTS

FOREWORD vi

PART 1: GUIDANCE DOCUMENT ON CHARACTERIZING AND COMMUNICATING UNCERTAINTY IN EXPOSURE ASSESSMENT

ACKNOWLEDGEMENTS viii

MEMBERS OF THE WHO/IPCS WORKING GROUP ON UNCERTAINTY IN
EXPOSURE ASSESSMENT ix

LIST OF ACRONYMS AND ABBREVIATIONS xi

EXECUTIVE SUMMARY xii

1. INTRODUCTION 1
 1.1 Why uncertainty analysis? 2
 1.2 Consideration of uncertainty in the harmonization of risk assessment methods 3
 1.3 Scope and objectives 3

2. CONTEXT, CONCEPTS AND DEFINITIONS 5
 2.1 Historical context and background 5
 2.2 Rationale for characterizing uncertainty in exposure assessment 6
  2.2.1 Assessment objectives 6
  2.2.2 Defining the conceptual exposure model 7
  2.2.3 Building an exposure model and assessment 8
 2.3 Planning for uncertainty analysis in exposure assessment 9
  2.3.1 Balancing the uncertainties of exposure and hazard 10
  2.3.2 Variability versus uncertainty 11
  2.3.3 Sensitivity analysis 13

3. SOURCES OF UNCERTAINTY 15
 3.1 Approaches and steps in exposure assessment 15
 3.2 Nature of uncertainty sources 16
  3.2.1 Scenario uncertainty 17
  3.2.2 Model uncertainty 18
  3.2.3 Parameter uncertainty 23

4. TIERED APPROACH TO UNCERTAINTY ANALYSIS 30
 4.1 Regulatory background 30
 4.2 Determination of the tiered level 31
  4.2.1 Tier 0 (screening) uncertainty analysis 31
  4.2.2 Tier 1 (qualitative) uncertainty analysis 32
  4.2.3 Tier 2 (deterministic) uncertainty analysis 33
  4.2.4 Tier 3 (probabilistic) uncertainty analysis 33

4.3 Summary of the tiered approach 36

5. UNCERTAINTY CHARACTERIZATION METHODS, INTERPRETATION AND USE 38
   5.1 Qualitative uncertainty characterization 38
      5.1.1 Rationale and objective 38
      5.1.2 Methodology for qualitative uncertainty characterization 39
      5.1.3 Conclusion 46
   5.2 Quantitative uncertainty characterization 46
      5.2.1 Intervals and probability bounds 47
      5.2.2 Fuzzy methods 48
      5.2.3 Probabilistic methods 49
      5.2.4 Sensitivity analysis 58
   5.3 Data and resource requirements 60
   5.4 Interpretation of results 61
   5.5 Use of uncertainty analysis in evaluation and validation 64
   5.6 Summary of uncertainty characterization methods 65

6. COMMUNICATION 67
   6.1 Introduction and historical background 67
   6.2 The position of exposure and uncertainty assessment in the risk communication process 69
      6.2.1 Uncertainty in exposure assessment as a prognostic technique 69
      6.2.2 From scenario definition to uncertainty analysis: communication with the risk managers 70
      6.2.3 Anticipating the demands of the audiences 73
      6.2.4 Requirements for accepted exposure assessment 74
   6.3 Proposals for the presentation/visualization of uncertainty 74
      6.3.1 Presentation of numerical results 75
      6.3.2 Communication of quantified uncertainties 76
      6.3.3 Communication of unquantified uncertainties 80
   6.4 Avoiding typical conflicts in risk communication 81
   6.5 Conclusions 83

7. CONCLUSIONS 84

8. REFERENCES 85

GLOSSARY OF TERMS 97

ANNEX 1: CASE-STUDY—QUALITATIVE UNCERTAINTY ANALYSIS 105
   A1.1 Introduction 105
   A1.2 Objective 105
   A1.3 Sources of uncertainty 105
   A1.4 Selected tier 106
   A1.5 Characterization and evaluation of uncertainty 106
   A1.6 Communication 108

    A1.6.1 Communication with other scientists 108
    A1.6.2 Communication with risk managers 109
    A1.6.3 Communication with the public 109
Appendix 1: Background for case-study 111

ANNEX 2: CASE-STUDY—QUANTITATIVE UNCERTAINTY ANALYSIS 119
A2.1 Introduction 119
A2.2 Methods used in the case-study 119
    A2.2.1 Conceptual model: the context, the question and scenario development 120
    A2.2.2 Modelling approach 121
    A2.2.3 Constructing input distributions 121
    A2.2.4 Variance propagation methods 122
A2.3 Case-study: PBLx exposure from fish ingestion 123
    A2.3.1 Elements of the exposure assessment: context and question 124
    A2.3.2 Scenario definition 124
    A2.3.3 Model selection 124
    A2.3.4 Parameter values and data 125
    A2.3.5 Worst-case scenario 128
    A2.3.6 Variance propagation 128
    A2.3.7 Variance propagation with uncertainty and variability combined 129
    A2.3.8 Variance propagation with uncertainty and variability separated 134
A2.4 Summary of the case-study 138

PART 2: HALLMARKS OF DATA QUALITY IN CHEMICAL EXPOSURE ASSESSMENT

PREPARATION OF THE DOCUMENT 140

1. INTRODUCTION 143

2. WHAT DO WE MEAN BY "DATA" IN EXPOSURE ASSESSMENT? 145

3. TOWARDS A BROADER DEFINITION OF QUALITY IN EXPOSURE ASSESSMENT: HALLMARKS OF DATA QUALITY 147
    3.1 Appropriateness 149
    3.2 Accuracy 150
    3.3 Integrity 151
    3.4 Transparency 153

4. FROM EXPOSURE DATA QUALITY TO THE QUALITY OF EXPOSURE ASSESSMENTS 155

5. CONCLUSIONS 157

6. REFERENCES 158

Harmonization Project Document No. 6

FOREWORD

Harmonization Project Documents are a family of publications by the World Health Organization (WHO) under the umbrella of the International Programme on Chemical Safety (IPCS) (WHO/ILO/UNEP). Harmonization Project Documents complement the Environmental Health Criteria (EHC) methodology (yellow cover) series of documents as authoritative documents on methods for the risk assessment of chemicals.

The main impetus for the current coordinated international, regional and national efforts on the assessment and management of hazardous chemicals arose from the 1992 United Nations Conference on Environment and Development (UNCED). UNCED Agenda 21, Chapter 19, provides the "blueprint" for the environmentally sound management of toxic chemicals. This commitment by governments was reconfirmed at the 2002 World Summit on Sustainable Development and in 2006 in the Strategic Approach to International Chemicals Management (SAICM). The IPCS project on the Harmonization of Approaches to the Assessment of Risk from Exposure to Chemicals (Harmonization Project) is conducted under Agenda 21, Chapter 19, and contributes to the implementation of SAICM. In particular, the project addresses the SAICM objective on Risk Reduction and the SAICM Global Plan of Action activity to "Develop and use new and harmonized methods for risk assessment".

The IPCS Harmonization Project goal is *to improve chemical risk assessment globally, through the pursuit of common principles and approaches, and, hence, strengthen national and international management practices that deliver better protection of human health and the environment within the framework of sustainability.* The Harmonization Project aims to harmonize global approaches to chemical risk assessment, including by developing international guidance documents on specific issues. The guidance is intended for adoption and use in countries and by international bodies in the performance of chemical risk assessments. The guidance is developed by engaging experts worldwide. The project has been implemented using a step-wise approach, first sharing information and increasing understanding of methods and practices used by various countries, identifying areas where convergence of different approaches would be beneficial and then developing guidance that enables implementation of harmonized approaches. The project uses a building block approach, focusing at any one time on the aspects of risk assessment that are particularly important for harmonization.

The project enables risk assessments (or components thereof) to be performed using internationally accepted methods, and these assessments can then be shared to avoid duplication and optimize use of valuable resources for risk management. It also promotes sound science as a basis for risk management decisions, promotes transparency in risk assessment and reduces unnecessary testing of chemicals. Advances in scientific knowledge can be translated into new harmonized methods.

This ongoing project is overseen by a geographically representative Harmonization Project Steering Committee and a number of ad hoc Working Groups that manage the detailed work. Finalization of documents includes a rigorous process of international peer review and public comment.

PART 1:
GUIDANCE DOCUMENT ON CHARACTERIZING AND COMMUNICATING UNCERTAINTY IN EXPOSURE ASSESSMENT

Part 1: Guidance Document on Characterizing and Communicating Uncertainty in Exposure Assessment

ACKNOWLEDGEMENTS

This Harmonization Project Document was prepared by the IPCS Working Group on Uncertainty in Exposure Assessment, under the chairmanship of Dr Gerhard Heinemeyer. The contribution of Dr Alexandre Zenié, including editing and compiling the public review draft document, is gratefully acknowledged.

MEMBERS OF THE WHO/IPCS WORKING GROUP ON UNCERTAINTY IN EXPOSURE ASSESSMENT

Listed below are the members of the WHO/IPCS Working Group on Uncertainty in Exposure Assessment who developed this document:

Dr Christiaan Delmaar
Centre for Substances and Integrated Risk Assessment (SIR), National Institute of Public Health and the Environment (RIVM), Bilthoven, Netherlands

Dr H. Christopher Frey
Professor, Department of Civil, Construction, and Environmental Engineering, North Carolina State University, Raleigh, NC, USA

Dr William C. Griffith
Associate Director, Institute for Risk Analysis and Risk Communication, Department of Environmental and Occupational Health Sciences, University of Washington, Seattle, WA, USA

Dr Andy Hart
Risk Analysis Team, Central Science Laboratory, Sand Hutton, York, United Kingdom

Dr Gerhard Heinemeyer (*Working Group Chair*)
Federal Institute for Risk Assessment, Berlin, Germany

Dr Roshini Jayewardene
Office of Chemical Safety, National Industrial Chemicals Notification & Assessment Scheme, Sydney, Australia

Dr Thomas E. McKone
Deputy Department Head, Indoor Environment Department, Lawrence Berkeley National Laboratory, Berkeley, CA, USA

Ms Bette Meek
Health Canada, Ottawa, Ontario, Canada

Dr Haluk Özkaynak
Senior Scientist, Environmental Protection Agency, Research Triangle Park, NC, United States of America (USA)

Dr Michael Schümann
Epidemiology Working Group, Department of Science and Health and Institute for Medical Biometry and Epidemiology (IMBE), Hamburg, Germany

Part 1: Guidance Document on Characterizing and Communicating Uncertainty in Exposure Assessment

Representatives of organizations

Dr Stephen Olin
Deputy Director, Research Foundation, International Life Sciences Institute, Washington, DC, USA

Ms Valérie Rolland (during development of the public review draft of the document)
Assistant Scientific Co-ordinator, Scientific Committee, European Food Safety Authority, Parma, Italy

Dr Alexandre Zenié
Institute for Health and Consumer Protection, Joint Research Centre, European Commission, Ispra, Italy

Secretariat

Ms Carolyn Vickers
International Programme on Chemical Safety, World Health Organization, Geneva, Switzerland

LIST OF ACRONYMS AND ABBREVIATIONS

1D	one-dimensional
2D	two-dimensional
ADI	acceptable daily intake
BCF	bioconcentration factor
bw	body weight
CCA	chromated copper arsenate
CDF	cumulative distribution function
CV	coefficient of variation
DPD	discrete probability distribution
EU	European Union
FAST	Fourier amplitude sensitivity test
GM	geometric mean
GSD	geometric standard deviation
IPCS	International Programme on Chemical Safety
K_{ow}	octanol–water partition coefficient
LHS	Latin hypercube sampling
LOAEL	lowest-observed-adverse-effect level
LOD	limit of detection
MC	Monte Carlo
NOAEL	no-observed-adverse-effect level
PBPK	physiologically based pharmacokinetic
REACH	Registration, Evaluation, Authorisation and Restriction of Chemicals
RfD	reference dose
SD	standard deviation
SHEDS	Stochastic Human Exposure and Dose Simulation
SOP	Standard Operating Procedure
TDI	tolerable daily intake
USA	United States of America
USEPA	United States Environmental Protection Agency
WHO	World Health Organization

Part 1: Guidance Document on Characterizing and Communicating Uncertainty in Exposure Assessment

EXECUTIVE SUMMARY

This guidance has been developed as a basis for transparently characterizing uncertainty in chemical exposure assessment to enable its full consideration in regulatory and policy decision-making processes. Uncertainties in exposure assessment are grouped under three categories—namely, parameter, model and scenario—with the guidance addressing both qualitative and quantitative descriptions. Guidance offered here is consistent with other projects addressing exposure in the WHO/IPCS Harmonization Project, including a monograph on *IPCS Risk Assessment Terminology*, which includes a glossary of key exposure assessment terminology, and a monograph on *Principles of Characterizing and Applying Human Exposure Models*.

The framework described in this monograph is considered applicable across a full range of chemical categories, such as industrial chemicals, pesticides, food additives and others. It is intended primarily for use by exposure assessors who are not intimately familiar with uncertainty analysis. The monograph aims to provide an insight into the complexities associated with characterizing uncertainties in exposure assessment and suggested strategies for incorporating them during human health risk assessments for environmental contaminants. This is presented in the context of comparability with uncertainties associated with hazard quantification in risk assessment.

This document recommends a tiered approach to the evaluation of uncertainties in exposure assessment using both qualitative and quantitative (both deterministic and probabilistic) methods, with the complexity of the analysis increasing as progress is made through the tiers. The report defines and identifies different sources of uncertainty in exposure assessment, outlines considerations for selecting the appropriate approach to uncertainty analysis as dictated by the specific objective and identifies the information needs of decision-makers and stakeholders. The document also provides guidance on ways to consider or characterize exposure uncertainties during risk assessment and risk management decision-making and on communicating the results. Illustrative examples based on environmental exposure and risk analysis case-studies are provided.

The monograph also recommends the adoption of 10 guiding principles for uncertainty analysis. These guiding principles are considered to be the general desirable goals or properties of good exposure assessment. They are mentioned in the text where most appropriate and are supported by more detailed recommendations for good practice. The 10 guiding principles are as follows:

1) Uncertainty analysis should be an integral part of exposure assessment.

2) The level of detail of the uncertainty analysis should be based on a tiered approach and consistent with the overall scope and purpose of the exposure and risk assessment.

3) Sources of uncertainty and variability should be systematically identified and evaluated in the exposure assessment.

4) The presence or absence of moderate to strong dependencies between model inputs is to be discussed and appropriately accounted for in the analysis.

5) Data, expert judgement or both should be used to inform the specification of uncertainties for scenarios, models and model parameters.

6) Sensitivity analysis should be an integral component of the uncertainty analysis in order to identify key sources of variability, uncertainty or both and to aid in iterative refinement of the exposure model.

7) Uncertainty analyses for exposure assessment should be documented fully and systematically in a transparent manner, including both qualitative and quantitative aspects pertaining to data, methods, scenarios, inputs, models, outputs, sensitivity analysis and interpretation of results.

8) The uncertainty analysis should be subject to an evaluation process that may include peer review, model comparison, quality assurance or comparison with relevant data or independent observations.

9) Where appropriate to an assessment objective, exposure assessments should be iteratively refined over time to incorporate new data, information and methods to better characterize uncertainty and variability.

10) Communication of the results of exposure assessment uncertainties to the different stakeholders should reflect the different needs of the audiences in a transparent and understandable manner.

Part 1: Guidance Document on Characterizing and Communicating Uncertainty in Exposure Assessment

1. INTRODUCTION

Individuals are exposed to a wide variety of chemicals in various indoor and outdoor microenvironments during the course of a typical day through inhalation, ingestion or dermal contact. *Exposure* is defined as contact between an *agent* and a *target*, where contact takes place on an *exposure surface* over an *exposure period* (Zartarian et al., 1997; IPCS, 2004). In the case of the present monograph, the agents of concern are chemical—although the World Health Organization (WHO)/International Programme on Chemical Safety (IPCS) Working Group considered the guidance to be also broadly applicable to other (physical and biological) agents. The targets are children, adults or sensitive subgroups in populations; the exposure surfaces are the external human boundaries (e.g. skin) or internal organs (e.g. gastrointestinal tract, lung surface); the exposure duration may be short (i.e. from minutes to hours to a day) or long (i.e. from days to months to a lifetime); and the health effects may be acute, intermittent or chronic. The process of estimating or measuring the magnitude, frequency and duration of exposure to an agent, along with the number and characteristics of the population exposed, is called an *exposure assessment*. In some health studies, the term "exposure assessment" may also include assessing the dose within the body after the agent enters the body via ingestion, inhalation or dermal absorption. This absorbed dose of the agent or its metabolite is also known as the *uptake*.

Historically, risk assessments have included four principal components: *hazard identification*,[1] or the identification of the type and nature of adverse effects that an agent has the inherent capacity to cause; *hazard characterization*, or the qualitative and, wherever possible, quantitative description of the inherent property of the agent of concern; *exposure assessment*, or the assessment of the magnitude of likely human exposures of an individual or a population to that agent; and *risk characterization*, or the qualitative and, wherever possible, quantitative determination of the probability of occurrence of adverse effects of the agent under defined exposure conditions. The entire risk assessment process is itself only one component of *risk analysis*, the other two being *risk management* and *risk communication*. Risk reduction is often achieved through exposure mitigation. Therefore, knowledge of the exposure is the basic prerequisite for risk characterization and for characterizing subsequent risk management strategies. The importance of exposure assessment is to provide information about the nature of the source and route of exposure and the individuals who are exposed. Risks cannot be reliably estimated if exposures and their uncertainties are not properly characterized and sufficiently quantified.

There are a number of aspects that must be taken into account in accurate estimation of exposure. Quantification of the magnitude and timing of personal exposures to agents of concern requires the identification of sources and media of concern, key exposure microenvironments, and routes and pathways of exposure that contribute most to an individual's exposure. Unfortunately, the information base on which to estimate emissions, concentrations, exposures and doses associated with each of these steps is sometimes completely lacking, frequently incomplete, not representative or otherwise uncertain. Given

---

[1] See the IPCS document on risk assessment terminology (IPCS, 2004). Important definitions are repeated in the text. Definitions of selected terms not included in IPCS (2004) are given in the Glossary of terms.

that complete information is never available, exposure assessors must make simplifying assumptions (e.g. use defaults) or rely on data that are not necessarily representative of the populations or conditions of interest (e.g. by extrapolating results that have been generated for other purposes). For example, concentrations of dioxins may be available for only one species of fish, so it may be necessary to extrapolate from these data to other species, if an estimate of overall exposure to dioxins from fish consumption is required.

Uncertainties in risk assessment include considerations related to missing, incomplete and/or incorrect knowledge, as well as those associated with ignorance and/or lack of awareness. Uncertainties should be characterized as transparently as possible to ensure their adequate consideration in decision-making concerning the need for and nature of appropriate risk management and communication.

Part 2 of this Harmonization Project Document is on data quality for chemical exposure assessment, because of its importance to the acceptance and credibility of the evaluation of uncertainty in an exposure analysis. Data quality for the purposes of this report deals with the completeness and clarity with which uncertainty is explained. This means that data with high uncertainty may be of high quality if the data and its uncertainty are clearly explained and carefully documented. A high-quality evaluation of uncertainty in an exposure analysis would provide the readers with the ability to re-evaluate all the choices and trade-offs made in the evaluation and to explore alternative choices and trade-offs. This is a difficult goal to achieve in most cases.

1.1 Why uncertainty analysis?

Uncertainty in risk assessment in the general sense is defined by IPCS (2004) as "imperfect knowledge concerning the present or future state of an organism, system, or (sub)population under consideration". In the context of exposure assessment, the exposures may be past, present or predicted future exposures, and the uncertainties in respect of each may differ. An adequate characterization of the uncertainties in exposure assessment is essential to the transparency of risk assessment and characterization of relevant data gaps to improve defensibility; it is also a critical basis for informed decision-making regarding the need for action to reduce risk and the nature of appropriate measures. Uncertainties should be considered explicitly in each step of the analysis and communicated throughout the process.

For exposure assessors, uncertainty analysis increases transparency and, thereby, the credibility of the process. Consequently, reliance on worst-case assumptions can be reduced and decision support improved. Uncertainty analysis also identifies important data gaps, which can be filled to improve the accuracy of estimation.

The consideration and expression of uncertainty are given particular attention in the Working Principles for Risk Analysis recently adopted by the Codex Alimentarius Commission (Codex, 2005: p. 104):

> 23. Constraints, uncertainties and assumptions having an impact on the risk assessment should be explicitly considered at each step in the risk assessment and documented in a transparent manner. Expression of uncertainty or variability in risk estimates may be qualitative or quantitative, but should be quantified to the extent that is scientifically achievable.

Part 1: Guidance Document on Characterizing and Communicating Uncertainty in Exposure Assessment

> ...
> 25. The report of the risk assessment should indicate any constraints, uncertainties, assumptions and their impact on the risk assessment. Minority opinions should also be recorded. The responsibility for resolving the impact of uncertainty on the risk management decision lies with the risk manager, not the risk assessors.

The rationale for characterizing uncertainty in exposure assessment is further described in section 2.2.

1.2 Consideration of uncertainty in the harmonization of risk assessment methods

Guidance to increased transparency in communicating uncertainty in exposure assessments contributes to the objectives of the IPCS Harmonization Project by promoting consistency in the presentation and defensibility of risk assessments. This includes increasing common understanding of the nature of information limitations that have an impact on the degree of confidence in the outcome of assessments and the resulting appropriate impact on associated management measures and research initiatives to address critical data gaps.

1.3 Scope and objectives

The objective of this monograph is to provide an overview on the nature and characterization of uncertainty in exposure assessments, including guidance on the identification of sources of uncertainty, its expression and application, not only in risk assessment, but also in risk management decisions, delineation of critical data gaps and communication to decision-makers and the public.

The content of this monograph is expected to be relevant to chemical regulators, the chemical industry and other stakeholders. It is intended to be applicable across the full range of chemical applications, including pesticides, food additives, industrial chemicals and by-products, and other contaminants.

Exposure analysts with varying levels of experience in uncertainty analysis are the specific intended audience for the monograph. The guidance provided in this monograph will enable exposure analysts to consider various aspects of uncertainty throughout the whole assessment, particularly when undertaking exposure assessments where uncertainty is identified as a significant problem.

However, since exposure assessment is an interdisciplinary activity, this monograph is also expected to be a useful resource for a wider audience, considering that each group may use the information contained herein for different purposes. The monograph provides an overview of the types of uncertainty encountered by an exposure analyst and provides guidance on how uncertainty can be characterized, analysed and described in a risk assessment and communicated effectively to a range of stakeholders.

The framework included herein provides for both qualitative and quantitative approaches to uncertainty analysis. It includes a tiered approach to methods for uncertainty analysis, the degree of quantitative analysis increasing with the complexity of assessment through each tier.

The monograph also aims to provide insight into the complexities associated with exposure assessments. The document considers "uncertainty analysis" in an inclusive manner and is not confined to statistical approaches alone.

The monograph:

- considers the context, concepts, definitions and issues in characterizing uncertainty in exposure assessment (chapter 2);
- identifies sources of uncertainty (chapter 3);
- outlines the tiered approach to characterization of uncertainty (chapter 4);
- describes qualitative and quantitative methods for characterizing uncertainty in exposure assessments (chapter 5);
- discusses issues relevant to effective communication of the outcome of the uncertainty analysis (chapter 6); and
- presents "guiding principles" for characterization of uncertainty in exposure assessment (throughout the report, where most appropriate).

Each chapter builds on the previous ones, and so chapters should be read in the order given to ensure complete understanding of the text. A glossary of terms is provided at the end of the chapters, followed by two annexes with case-studies to illustrate both qualitative (Annex 1) and quantitative (Annex 2) uncertainty analysis.

2. CONTEXT, CONCEPTS AND DEFINITIONS

This chapter provides the context, concepts and definitions related to uncertainty analysis in exposure assessment that are necessary to an understanding of subsequent chapters in the monograph.

2.1 Historical context and background

The complexity of exposure assessments necessarily varies, depending on their purpose. Quantitative approaches to exposure assessment have evolved over time as new methodologies have developed, which has led to increasing detail and transparency and the potential for greater harmony in the results obtained from different exposure models.

In early exposure assessments used in risk characterization, practitioners often used single point estimates of the maximum exposure of individuals to compare with measures of dose–response. Such estimates often lacked transparency in the context of the assumptions on which they were based and led to confusion in terminology (employing concepts such as "upper-bound exposure" and "maximally exposed individual").

The limited transparency of traditional exposure assessments has been an obstacle to harmonization. The use of simple bounding estimates in exposure assessment, for example, precluded harmonization among agencies using different bounding assumptions. The limited transparency also failed to provide decision-makers with important information relevant to risk characterization and risk management, such as the population distribution of exposures and uncertainties. As a result, the impact of critical data gaps and research priorities were often not clearly articulated, and transparency around the incorporated degree of conservatism was often insufficient. This may have resulted in less than optimum efficiency in allocation of resources to risk management versus data generation to better inform the characterization of risks.

More recently, there has been increasing emphasis on the characterization of the exposure of different individuals in the population. For example, the United States Environmental Protection Agency's (USEPA) guidelines for exposure assessment, issued in 1992, called for both high-end and central tendency estimates for the population (USEPA, 1992). The high end was considered as that which could occur for the 90th percentile or higher of exposed individuals, and the central tendency might represent an exposure somewhere near the median or mean of the distribution of exposed individuals.

Through the 1990s, there has been increasing emphasis also on characterization of the distinction between interindividual variability and uncertainty in exposure assessments (e.g. NRC, 1994). During this time, there was also growing interest and use of probabilistic simulation methods, such as those based on Monte Carlo (see below) or closely related methods, as the basis for estimating differences in exposures among individuals or, in some cases, in estimating the uncertainty associated with any particular exposure estimate (USEPA, 1997b).

These converging developments have brought the field of probabilistic exposure assessment from the background to a central part of exposure assessment today in many applications. The transparency afforded by probabilistic characterization and separation of uncertainty and variability in exposure assessment (see section 2.3.2 below) offers potential benefits in the context of increasing common understanding as a basis for greater convergence in methodology.

The historical context of uncertainty estimation in exposure assessment can be traced to the convergence of developments in multiple disciplines. For example, Stanislaw Ulam and John von Neumann are typically credited with creation of the Monte Carlo method for simulation of random events in 1946 (see Metropolis & Ulam, 1949; Eckhardt, 1987). However, a paper by Lord Kelvin in 1901 appears to apply concepts similar to Monte Carlo to a discussion of the Boltzmann equation, and there are other precedents (Kelvin, 1901). The modern incarnation of Monte Carlo was first used for prediction of neutron release during nuclear fission and has since been applied in a wide variety of disciplines.

2.2 Rationale for characterizing uncertainty in exposure assessment

Decision-makers and stakeholders typically ask a variety of questions about exposure. These questions motivate both the structure of the exposure assessment and the need for uncertainty analysis in that assessment. They include the following:

- What is the distribution of exposures among different members of an exposed population?
- How precise are the exposure estimates?
- How precise do the exposure estimates need to be?
- What is the pedigree of the numbers used as input to an exposure assessment?
- What are the key sources of uncertainty in the exposure assessment?
- How should efforts be targeted to improve the precision of the exposure estimates?
- How significant are differences between two alternatives?
- How significant are apparent trends over time?
- How effective are proposed control or management strategies?
- Is there a systematic error (bias) in the estimates? Is there ongoing research that might fill critical data gaps within the near term?
- Are the estimates based upon measurements, modelling or expert judgement?

To address these questions, an exposure assessment should begin with a definition of the assessment objective (section 2.2.1). From this follows the need to define and evaluate the conceptual exposure model (section 2.2.2). The goal of the conceptual model is to establish exposure links via exposure pathways to exposure routes and relative magnitude of uptake or intake by different exposure routes. These questions are discussed in more detail in section 5.4 with respect to interpretation of the results of a probabilistic exposure assessment.

2.2.1 Assessment objectives

Exposure assessments provide important inputs to risk assessments and other health studies. Although the discussions here are broadly relevant to exposure assessments, our particular focus is on the objectives defined by risk assessment. Risk assessment includes the following four steps: (1) hazard identification, (2) hazard characterization, (3) exposure assessment and (4) risk characterization. Uncertainty is inherent to each of these steps and can accumulate as one moves from one step to the next. In the exposure step, uncertainty arises from insufficient knowledge about relevant exposure scenarios, exposure models and model inputs.

The ultimate goal of exposure assessment is to be able to link sources of, for example, pollutants to the concentration of the agents with which people come into contact, to exposure, uptake and dose in the target population group and to biological changes or effects that may lead to adverse health outcomes. Understanding these linkages and being able to measure and model the linkages and the impacts through exposure assessment are vital to scientific and public health policy evaluations.

In conducting an exposure assessment, analysts are often challenged to address a number of technical questions, such as:

- Are the measurement data and/or the modelling estimates actually representative of the target group—either the general population or a selected sensitive subgroup?
- How many measurement data are needed to represent the vulnerable population, such as children or the elderly?
- How do we extrapolate from a relatively small sample to the larger group?
- Does the exposure model capture the important exposure pathways and routes, and does it quantify the exposures reliably?
- Do the assessments also describe the variability and uncertainty associated with the exposure scenarios or processes, so that a user understands any limitations of exposures and risk estimates?

Performing a qualitative or a quantitative variability and/or uncertainty analysis is often at the heart of addressing such important issues.

Exposure assessment, however, is a highly complex process having different levels of uncertainties, with qualitative and quantitative consequences. Exposure assessors must consider many different types of sources of exposures, the physical, chemical and biological characteristics of substances that influence their fate and transport in the environment and their uptake, individual mobility and behaviours, and different exposure routes and pathways, among others. These complexities make it important to begin with a clear definition of the conceptual model and a focus on how uncertainty and variability play out as one builds from the conceptual model towards the mathematical/statistical model.

2.2.2 Defining the conceptual exposure model

As pointed out in the WHO/IPCS monograph entitled *Principles of Characterizing and Applying Human Exposure Models* (IPCS, 2005b), the first step of an exposure analysis is to establish a *conceptual model*, which maps out a framework designed to reflect the links between the pollutant source and the contact for human exposure and its processes. The conceptual model helps to define the physical, chemical and behavioural information and exposure algorithms by which the resulting mathematical/statistical model captures actual exposure scenarios.

In Figure 1, a conceptual model of exposure to formaldehyde is given. It shows where formaldehyde comes from, sources of its release and pathways of exposure to it.

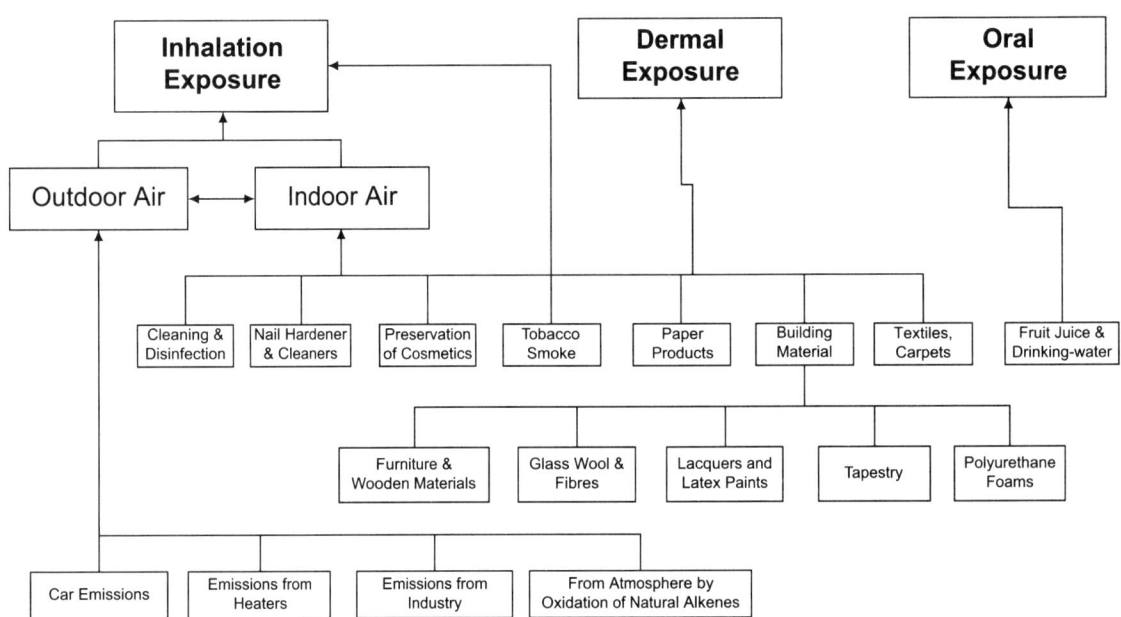

Figure 1: Example of a conceptual model of exposure—Formaldehyde (adapted from Heinemeyer et al., 2006)

Scenarios may be defined under the umbrella of this conceptual model. There are different levels of scenarios, such as that describing the release of formaldehyde from furniture. Each of the exposures from one of the sources may be characterized by a particular scenario, but all of these scenarios may be combined to yield bigger and more complex scenarios, such as the inhalation exposure pathway. In this concept, the scenario describing the whole exposure including all sources and paths represents a very complex construction.

2.2.3 Building an exposure model and assessment

An exposure assessment, which, according to IPCS (2004), is the process of estimating or measuring the magnitude, frequency and duration of exposure to an agent, along with the number and characteristics of the population exposed, is based on the following three elements: "scenario", "model" and "parameter". An exposure scenario provides the basis for building a mathematical model (algorithm). WHO defines the term *exposure scenario* as "a combination of facts, assumptions, and inferences that define a discrete situation where potential exposures may occur. These may include the source, the exposed population, the time frame of exposure, microenvironment(s), and activities. Scenarios are often created to aid exposure assessors in estimating exposure" (IPCS, 2004). According to the conceptual scenario, a model can be simple or complex. Based on the formaldehyde example above, a model can describe the oral intake of juice having a certain formaldehyde content, or it can describe the complex migration and release of formaldehyde from a polyurethane foam and its further distribution into room air with subsequent inhalation exposure. The combination of all the above-mentioned sources of formaldehyde may also lead to complexity in the mathematical model.

The term *model* is used to describe exposure including all the circumstances, the scenarios and their mathematical expressions. The term model is also used for computer programs to calculate exposure. In clinical pharmacology, a model characterizes the mathematical expression of the uptake, distribution and elimination of a drug from the body. WHO defines *exposure model* as "a conceptual or mathematical representation of the exposure process" (IPCS, 2004). This means that the model includes both concept and mathematical description of the exposure process.

The term *parameter* has several different meanings, ranging from specific to general. An example of the specific meaning of the term is a constant in a function that determines the specific form of the function but not its general nature. For example, the parameters of a normal distribution are the mean and standard deviation. These parameters have constant values for a particular population distribution. In practice, parameters of models are often calibrated (e.g. parameters of a regression model that is fitted to data) or may be physical constants (e.g. octanol–water partition coefficient, or K_{ow}). However, many practitioners use the word parameter synonymously with any input to a model, whether it is a true constant, a calibrated constant or a variable. In this document, the term parameter is used in a general sense and is often inclusive of physical constants, calibration constants and other inputs to a model that may vary, such as over time, over space or among individuals in an exposed population.

2.3 Planning for uncertainty analysis in exposure assessment

Because the objective of an exposure assessment is to characterize both the magnitude and the reliability of exposure scenarios, planning for an uncertainty analysis is a key element of an exposure assessment. The aims of the uncertainty analysis in this context are to individually and jointly characterize and quantify the exposure prediction uncertainties resulting from each step of the analysis. In performing an uncertainty analysis, typically the main sources of uncertainties are first characterized qualitatively and then quantified using a tiered approach (see chapter 4). In general, exposure uncertainty analyses attempt to differentiate between key sources of uncertainties: scenario uncertainties, model uncertainties and parameter uncertainties (for definitions, see section 3.2).

In exposure assessment, uncertainty arises from insufficient knowledge about relevant exposure scenarios, exposure models and model inputs. Each of these sources of uncertainty has factors that determine the magnitude of uncertainty and variation. For example, Mosbach-Schulz (1999) identified three factors related to the uncertainty and variability of input data:

namely, diversity, variation and statistical uncertainty. *Diversity* is related to the real differences among groups of substances and individuals (e.g. age, sex). *Variation* describes existing differences within each group (e.g. behavioural, anthropometric). *Statistical uncertainty* encompasses that fraction of variability that is a result of given sample sizes (statistical errors of the estimates). Additional uncertainty with respect to samples might result from restrictions towards the degree of representativity and deviations in the degree from differential participation of subgroups, which might raise concern about systematic bias. Measurement error (especially in data from questionnaires), regional and temporal variance as well as aggregation bias (using average habits and consumption) might contribute to uncertainty.

2.3.1 Balancing the uncertainties of exposure and hazard

The extent of accommodation and characterization of uncertainty in exposure assessment must necessarily be balanced against similar considerations with respect to hazard, since the outcome of any risk assessment is a function of comparison of the two. If, for example, there is limited information to inform quantitatively on hazard and, as a result, a need to rely on defaults, there is limited benefit to be gained in developing the exposure analysis such that any increase in certainty is cancelled by uncertainties of greater magnitude associated with quantification of critical hazard, as a basis for a complete risk assessment.

Often, estimates of exposure are compared directly with benchmark doses or concentrations (i.e. those that result in a critical effect of defined increase in incidence, such as 5% or 10%). Alternatively, they are compared with either a *lowest-observed-adverse-effect level* (LOAEL), the lowest concentration that leads to an adverse effect, or *no-observed-adverse-effect level* (NOAEL), the highest concentration that does not lead to an adverse effect, or their equivalents. This results in a "*margin of safety*" or "*margin of exposure*". Alternatively, estimates of exposure are compared with tolerable or reference concentrations or doses, which are based on the division of benchmark doses and/or concentrations or the NOAELs or LOAELs by factors that account for uncertainties in the available data.

The NOAEL or benchmark dose/concentration is selected, then, generally to be at or below the threshold in animals; uncertainty factors are then applied to estimate the subthreshold in *sensitive human* populations, with a 10-fold default factor addressing interspecies differences (i.e. the variation in response between animals and a representative healthy human population) and another 10-fold factor accounting for interindividual variability in humans (the variation in response between a representative healthy human population and sensitive subgroups). While additional factors are sometimes applied to account for deficiencies of the database, the 100-fold default value is common.

Division of benchmark doses and/or effect levels by default uncertainty factors represents the lower end of a continuum of increasingly data-informed approaches to estimation of hazard. For example, where additional adequate quantitative data on interspecies differences or human variability in either toxicokinetics or toxicodynamics (mode of action) are available, *chemical-specific adjustment factors* provide for their incorporation to replace appropriately weighted components of default uncertainty factors. This requires subdivision of default uncertainty factors for interspecies differences and interindividual variation into toxicokinetic and toxicodynamic components (IPCS, 2005a).

Physiologically based pharmacokinetic (PBPK) modelling sometimes constitutes a basis for replacement of default components of uncertainty for toxicokinetics and a portion of toxicodynamics. Where data are sufficient, a full biologically based dose–response model addresses additional uncertainties with respect to both interspecies differences and interindividual variability in both kinetics and dynamics.

As the extent of data and complexity of the analysis along this continuum increases, approaches are often presented probabilistically, including sensitivity analysis. For example, consideration is given to the probabilistic presentation of default uncertainty factors as a basis for development of reference or tolerable concentrations and/or doses or margins of safety or exposure, based on the fraction of the population to be protected.

The extent of development and characterization of uncertainty associated with estimating exposure should take into account the nature of quantification of hazard in any risk assessment to ensure comparability of the two.

2.3.2 Variability versus uncertainty

Exposure assessment informs decision-making regarding protection of human health.

As Cullen and Frey (1999) point out, decision-making regarding control of exposures is typically aimed at protecting a particular group, such as the entire population of a country, a highly exposed subpopulation, random individuals within a population or specific individuals with a particular characteristic in common, such as children. As pointed out by NRC (1994), there is certainty that different individuals will have different exposures. For example, each individual may have a different behavioural (activity) pattern, dietary pattern and physiological characteristics (e.g. breathing rates). For a given individual, these can change over time; at any given time, these vary between individuals. These differences lead to *variability* in the exposure levels of the individuals.

However, the true exposures are rarely known for a given individual and are estimated using modelling procedures based upon available data. Uncertainty regarding exposure estimates arises as a result of the limited availability of empirical information, as well as limitations in the measurements, models or techniques used to develop representations of complex physical, chemical and biological processes. As described by NRC (1994), "uncertainty forces decision makers to judge how probable it is that risks will be overestimated or underestimated for every member of the exposed population". Furthermore, because every individual can have a different exposure level, it is also possible that the estimate of uncertainty can differ among individuals.

Thus, the notions of intraindividual variability and uncertainty are distinct concepts, because they arise for different reasons. Variability is an inherent property of the system being modelled. In contrast, uncertainty can be conceptualized as dependent on the current state of knowledge regarding the system being modelled. From this perspective, uncertainty is more a property of the data than it is of the system being modelled. For example, the ability to make predictions regarding exposure will depend on the data and models available at the time that the prediction is made. Over time, perhaps "better" data might become available. Data could be considered better if they are more representative, more precise or both. A model would be better than another if it had less systematic error and greater precision. As the quality of data and models improves, the amount of uncertainty inherent in a prediction decreases. Thus, uncertainty is reduced as the result of developing an improved knowledge base.

Two important considerations in probabilistic exposure assessment are whether to quantify uncertainty and whether to separate it from variability within the analysis and output:

- When *only variability* is quantified, the output is a single distribution representing a "best estimate" of variation in exposure. This can be used to estimate exposure for different percentiles of the population but provides no confidence intervals and may give a false impression of certainty.

- When input distributions representing *variability and uncertainty are combined* (e.g. by "one-dimensional" or 1D Monte Carlo), the output is again a single distribution, but now represents a mixture of variability and uncertainty (and is therefore wider; see Figure 2). It can be interpreted as an uncertainty distribution for the exposure of a *single member of the population selected at random*. This can be used to read off the probability of a randomly chosen individual being exposed to any given level.

- When *variability and uncertainty are propagated separately* (e.g. by "two-dimensional" or 2D Monte Carlo), they can be shown separately in the output. For example, the output can be presented as three cumulative curves: a central one representing the median estimate of the distribution for variation in exposure, and two outer ones representing lower and upper confidence bounds for the distribution (Figure 2). This can be used to read off exposure estimates for different percentiles of the population, together with confidence bounds showing the combined effect of those uncertainties that have been quantified.

Strategy or approach is then determined by the desired nature of the output: an estimate for a given percentile of the population with (option 3) or without (option 1) confidence bounds, or the probability of a randomly chosen individual falling below (or above) a given exposure (option 2).

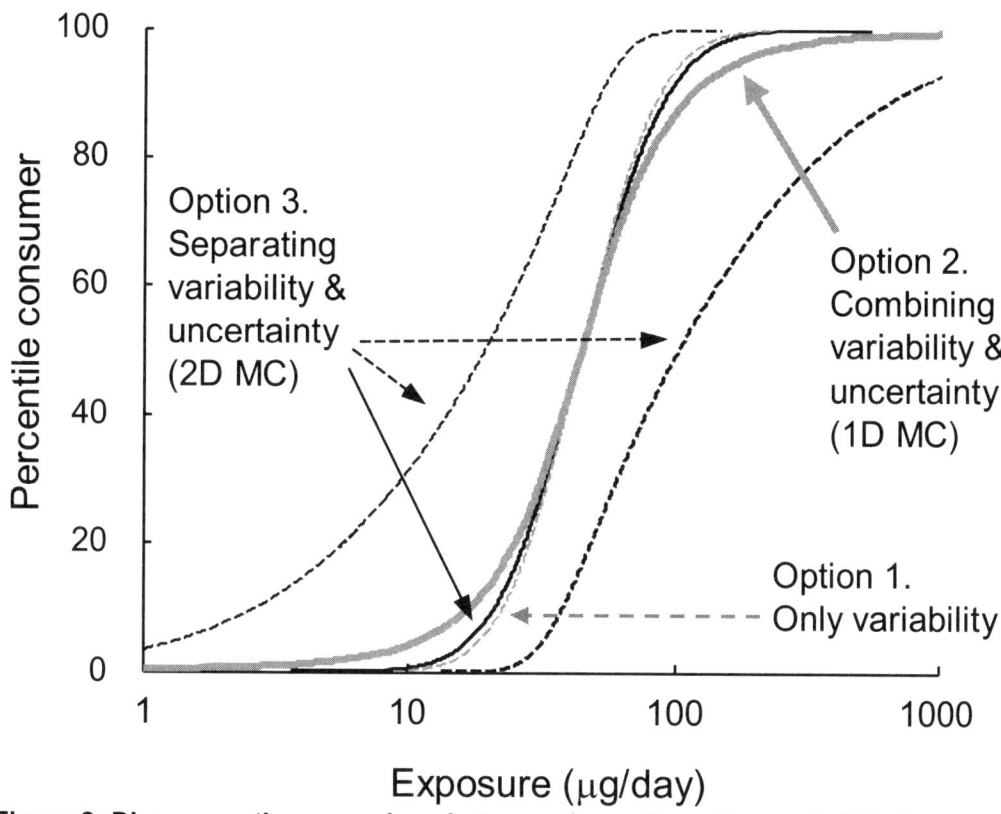

Figure 2: Diagrammatic comparison between three alternative probabilistic approaches for the same exposure assessment. In option 1, only variability is quantified. In option 2, both variability and uncertainty are propagated together. In option 3, variability and uncertainty are propagated separately. MC = Monte Carlo.

2.3.3 Sensitivity analysis

Sensitivity analysis is the study of how the variation in the outputs of a model can be attributed to, qualitatively or quantitatively, different sources of variation in model inputs or structural differences among alternative scenarios or models. Saltelli et al. (2000) and Mokhtari & Frey (2005) provide detailed overviews of sensitivity analysis. Sensitivity analysis is most commonly applied to assess the effect of variations in one or more model inputs on variation in a model output. Sensitivity analysis provides a tool to identify the inputs of greatest importance by (1) quantifying the impact of changes in values of one or more model inputs on a model output, (2) evaluating how variation in model output values can be apportioned among model inputs and (3) identifying which inputs and what values of such inputs contribute the most to best or worst outcomes of interest (e.g. low or high exposures).

Sensitivity analysis can answer a number of key questions, such as the following:

- What is the impact of changes in input values on model output?
- What are the key controllable sources of variability?
- What are the key contributors to the output uncertainty?

- How can variation in output values be apportioned among model inputs?
- What are the ranges of inputs associated with best or worst outcomes?
- What are the critical limits for controllable sources of variability that will lead to achievement of risk management goals?

A controllable source of variability is also known as a critical control point and refers to a point, step or procedure at which control can be applied and a hazard can be prevented, eliminated or reduced to an acceptable level. A critical limit is a criterion that must be met for each preventive measure associated with a controllable source of variability or critical control point.

Sensitivity analysis can be used to identify and prioritize key sources of uncertainty or variability. Knowledge of key sources of uncertainty and their relative importance to the assessment end-point is useful in determining whether additional data collection or research would be useful in an attempt to reduce uncertainty. If uncertainty can be reduced in an important model input, then the corresponding uncertainty in the model output would also be reduced. Knowledge of key sources of controllable variability, their relative importance and critical limits is useful in developing risk management options.

Sensitivity analysis is useful not only because it provides insight for a decision-maker, but also because it assists a model developer in identifying which assumptions and inputs matter the most to the estimate of the assessment end-point. Therefore, sensitivity analysis can be used during model development to identify priorities for data collection, as well as to determine which inputs matter little to the assessment and thus need not be a significant focus of time or other resources. Furthermore, insights obtained from sensitivity analysis can be used to determine which parts of a model might be the focus of further refinement, such as efforts to develop more detailed empirical or mechanistic relationships to better explain variability. Thus, sensitivity analysis is recommended as a tool for prioritizing model development activities.

3. SOURCES OF UNCERTAINTY

Uncertainties arise in various stages of exposure assessment. These uncertainties should be confronted as an integral part of the process, rather than being limited to the final stage.

> **Principle 1**
>
> *Uncertainty analysis should be an integral part of exposure assessment.*

The level of detail of the assessment may vary greatly, depending on the purpose for which it is carried out (i.e. as a screening-level assessment or as a detailed, probabilistic assessment). The level of detail with which the uncertainty is analysed will vary accordingly and should, as a rule, be consistent with the level of detail of the exposure assessment.

The objective of an uncertainty analysis is to determine differences in the output of the assessment due to the combined uncertainties in the inputs and to identify and characterize key sources of uncertainty. To this end, a first step in the treatment of the uncertainty in an exposure study consists of the identification of the sources of uncertainty that are relevant for the study.

There are numerous methods for the subsequent qualitative and quantitative characterization of the relevant uncertainties. These methods are covered in sections 5.1 and 5.2, respectively.

This chapter gives an overview of different sources of uncertainty that may arise at different stages of the exposure assessment. Therefore, this chapter aims to systematically describe the steps of exposure assessment and the related sources of uncertainties.

Section 3.1 provides a brief overview of approaches and steps typically used in exposure assessment. Next, in section 3.2, a taxonomy of the different sources of uncertainty is given. There are numerous texts providing schemes for the classification of sources of uncertainty. The classification given below follows in outline the one given in the USEPA's *Guidelines for Exposure Assessment* (USEPA, 1992).

> **Principle 2**
>
> *The level of detail of the uncertainty analysis should be based on a tiered approach and consistent with the overall scope and purpose of the exposure and risk assessment.*

3.1 Approaches and steps in exposure assessment

Exposure assessment uses a wide array of techniques and information sources. The approaches to exposure assessment can be classified into four general categories:

1) the use of professional (i.e. expert) judgement alone, with no attempt to use the direct or indirect approaches described below, to arrive at a qualitative assessment of the

magnitude of exposure, i.e. "significant exposure is not expected from a small deviation of a specific value";

2) direct approaches to quantify the exposure being assessed, using monitoring data from real-life situations;
3) indirect approaches to quantify the exposure being assessed, using simulation and real-life modelling; and
4) combined or hybrid approaches to quantify the exposure being assessed, using both direct and indirect methods.

Common to all approaches are the following working steps:

- specification of the purpose and scope of the assessment; and
- building of the assessment scenario.

In addition, the quantitative approaches include:

- a description of the selected assessment approach, including monitoring and/or modelling steps, which specify the parameters needed in the assessment;
- selection of data and specification of any assumptions;
- execution of calculations; and
- documentation, interpretation and presentation of results.

3.2 Nature of uncertainty sources

Uncertainty is the lack of knowledge of vital parts that are needed to perform an exposure assessment. Uncertainty can, at least in principle, be reduced by research to obtain necessary or applicable information or data.

Uncertainty pertains to different steps and approaches in the assessment. It can be classified into three broad categories:

1) *Scenario uncertainty*: Uncertainty in specifying the exposure scenario that is consistent with the scope and purpose of the assessment.
2) *Model uncertainty*: Uncertainty due to gaps in scientific knowledge that hamper an adequate capture of the correct causal relations between exposure factors.
3) *Parameter uncertainty*: Uncertainty involved in the specification of numerical values (be they point values or distributions of values) for the factors that determine the exposure.

Classification using the three categories defined above is not as strict as it may seem, and the uncertainties may in practice arise in overlapping areas. For instance, numerical values of model parameters are often determined from the calibration of a model against some data set. In this case, the parameter values may be uncertain to the extent both that this calibration data set suffers from uncertainty in measurement (parameter uncertainty) and that the model that is calibrated is not adequate for the situation (model uncertainty).

A clear decision as to whether the uncertainty is related to the scenario, model or parameters is sometimes difficult. There are, as mentioned, overlaps, and even expert opinions may deviate. Identification of the sources of scenario uncertainty is a matter of interpretation and depends on the clarity with which the scope and purpose of the assessment are given.

It is not possible to quantify all sources of uncertainty. Therefore, expression of uncertainty, variability or both in exposure estimates may be qualitative or quantitative, but uncertainty should be quantified to the extent that is scientifically achievable. The concepts of variability and uncertainty are distinct, and typically there will be a need to distinguish these based upon the problem formulation.

> **Principle 3**
>
> *Sources of uncertainty and variability should be systematically identified and evaluated in the exposure assessment.*

3.2.1 Scenario uncertainty

A sound description of the scenario is an important prerequisite for modelling exposure or for interpreting measured exposure data. The description of the scenario governs the choice of the model and that of model variables (model parameters). The scenario description can be divided into several parts:

- a description of the source of the chemical;
- the characteristics of the release of the chemical to the contacting environment, the distribution of the substance in that volume and its disappearance from that volume; and
- in any case of exposure analysis, a calculation of the amount of the substance that will enter the body using the concentration of the substance in the contacting medium (i.e. in air, on skin or in media that can be eaten or swallowed) and an uptake rate (i.e. respiration rate, dermal absorption rate or consumption rate).

Also, behavioural data are important for characterizing the exposure route, the frequencies of use/consumption and the duration of use/consumption.

Scenario uncertainty includes descriptive errors (e.g. wrong or incomplete information), aggregation errors (e.g. approximations for volume and time), errors of assessment (e.g. choice of the wrong model) and errors of incomplete analysis (e.g. overlooking an important exposure pathway).

Scenario uncertainty characterization may include a description of the information used for the scenario characterization (scenario definition). This includes a description of the purpose of the exposure analysis. For regulatory purposes, the level of the tiered approach is essential to describe the choice of data, whether defaults, upper-bound estimates or other single point estimates, or distributions have been used. This choice may govern the kind of uncertainty analysis.

The definition of the scope and purpose of each exposure assessment provides the specifications for building the exposure scenario, which represents the real-life situation that is to be assessed and provides the boundary limits of the assessment. As pointed out previously, the scenario uncertainty includes the "facts, assumptions and inferences" that are taken into consideration and used, but, in reality, are not actually representative of the scope and purpose of the assessment. These sources of uncertainty typically include incomplete and/or non-relevant specification of the following:

- agent to be considered;
- exposed populations;
- spatial and temporal information (e.g. geographic applicability and seasonal applicability);
- microenvironments;
- population activities;
- sources of the released agent;
- exposure pathways;
- exposure events;
- exposure routes; and
- risk management measures.

Incomplete and irrelevant specification of the above elements of the exposure scenario may be related to lack of knowledge, descriptive errors, aggregation errors, errors in professional judgement and incomplete analysis (USEPA, 1992).

The following short descriptions represent examples that were primarily referred to as scenario uncertainties.

Examples of scenario uncertainties:

1. Lack of prior knowledge of coffee as an important source of acrylamide exposure
2. Lack of consideration of the dermal pathway in the assessment of exposure to insecticide sprays
3. Lack of consideration of dust as an important carrier in the assessment of a non-volatile ingredient of a home insecticide
4. Characterization of room air concentrations without consideration of air exchange

---

3.2.2 Model uncertainty

In exposure assessments, mathematical and statistical models are often applied to represent the entire exposure process or parts of it. Models used in this sense quantitatively describe the relationship between their input parameters and the responses of the entire system (or part of it) to changes in these inputs. To a certain extent, a model is always a simplification of reality. The level of detail with which a model describes a system should be consistent with the objective of the assessment.

Model uncertainty is principally based upon (1) modelling errors (i.e. non-consideration of parameters) and (2) relation (dependency) errors (i.e. drawing incorrect conclusions from correlations). For example, the mathematical formula of a model describing the concentration–time curve of a substance emitted from, for example, glue should consider an algorithm that describes the time-dependent increase of the substance in a room, its distribution and the decrease of the concentration. Body weight correlates non-linearly with body surface, which may lead to dependency errors when, for example, extrapolating exposures from adults to children.

In using models, the following sources of uncertainty are to be considered:

- linking the selected conceptual model to the adopted scenario (model boundaries);
- model dependencies;
- model assumptions;
- model detail (i.e. simple or complex);
- model extrapolation; and
- model implementation and technical model aspects (e.g. errors in software and hardware).

Examples of some of these sources of uncertainty are given below, and further details are provided in section 5.1.

3.2.2.1 Model boundaries: Representation of the adopted scenario

The scope and purpose of the exposure assessment inform the formulation of one or more scenarios for which exposures are to be estimated. The exposure estimation approach should be capable of faithfully representing the key structural assumptions of the scenario, such as exposed population, agents to be considered, spatial and temporal scope, microenvironments and so on (see section 3.2.1 for a complete list). If the modelling approach omits any of the relevant elements, then the estimates could be biased. If the modelling approach includes irrelevant, unnecessary or superfluous elements, then, at best, the model is likely to be more cumbersome to deal with than it needs to be, or, at worst, biases may be introduced.

The development or selection of a model involves decisions regarding the time, space, number of chemicals, etc., used in guiding modelling of the system. Risks can be understated or overstated if the model boundary is misspecified. For example, if a study area is defined to be too large and includes a significant number of low-exposure areas, then a population-level risk distribution can be diluted by including less-exposed individuals, which can, in turn, result in a risk-based decision that does not sufficiently protect the most-exposed individuals in the study area. A common challenge in exposure modelling is to achieve the proper representation of averaging times for exposures when considering all model inputs and to account for the proper geographic scope of sources of agents, microenvironments and human activity.

3.2.2.2 Dependency errors

Dependency errors arise from lack of consideration of dependencies between parameters (be it by mistake or as a simplifying assumption) or incorrect inference of dependencies between parameters. For instance, anthropometric properties such as body weight, dermal surfaces and inhalation rate are correlated. Not including empirically proven correlations in a probabilistic assessment will yield incorrect exposure estimates.

> **Examples of dependency errors:**
>
> 1. Failure to account for possible correlation between the frequency of use of a consumer product by a consumer and the amount used per use.
> 2. Expression of a linear relation by taking an exponential term.
> 3. Using a constant emission rate to describe the evaporation of a chemical from a matrix without taking into account that the rate of evaporation will depend on the chemical concentration in both air and the matrix.
> 4. In simulating lifelong exposure to a persistent pollutant, the body weight of a simulated individual at different stages of life will be correlated. If a person is heavy as an adolescent, there is a decreased probability that he or she will be a lighter-than-average adult. Not taking this dependency into account may lead to unrealistic evaluations.
> 5. Failure to account for dependency of body weight and breathing volume. The inhalation rate (Q_{inh}) depends on the basic metabolic rate (BMR) of humans by the equation:
>
> $$Q_{inh} = BMR \times H \times VQ$$
>
> where:
>
> H = oxygen uptake,
> VQ = ventilation equivalent.
>
> On the other hand, the BMR depends on body weight (BW) as follows:
>
> $$BMR = BW \times CF + C$$
>
> where CF is the correlation factor and C a numerical constant (Layton, 1993).
>
> This leads to the relation of inhalation rate and body weight, expressed as:
>
> $$Q_{inh} = (BW \times CF + C) \times H \times VQ$$

3.2.2.3 Alternative model assumptions

Different models can be built based on different scientific assumptions when the correct assumptions are unclear and cannot be asserted (e.g. the form of regression in regression models, the appropriate number and type of compartments and their connections in a compartmental model).

> **Example of alternative model assumptions:**
>
> A number of skin absorption models have been described, all of them using physicochemical properties of the substances (e.g. molecular weight, log K_{ow}) as the most important delimiters (Fiserova-Bergerova et al., 1990). Usually the rate of absorption per area will be estimated. In simple exposure models, however, the absorption is simply expressed by a fraction (i.e. an estimated absorbed percentage of the total amount of the substance).

3.2.2.4 Model detail

A model is a hypothesis regarding how a system works or responds to changes in its inputs. The development of a model involves decisions regarding what to include (or exclude) in the model and how much to aggregate the representation of processes that are included in the scope of the model. For example, a decision might be made to exclude a specific exposure pathway from a model because it is deemed to be of negligible impact to total exposures from all pathways. A decision might be made to aggregate, combine or lump two or more agents into a single generic chemical species (e.g. several specific aldehydes might be treated generically as one chemical group).

Simplifying assumptions in model development can be made for reasons of tractability and transparency or because of a lack of knowledge of the correct model structure or system parameters—for instance, modelling the indoor air concentration assuming well mixed air conditions in the room versus including a description of the dispersion of the chemical through the room air, or the aggregation of several compartments of a PBPK model into one compartment. Simplifications of a model may limit the extent of the model domain or yield results with a higher degree of uncertainty, which may or may not be acceptable in view of the objective of the exposure assessment.

Example of model detail:

Simple model

A very simple worst-case model to estimate the room air concentration resulting from the release of a chemical would, for example, neglect the details of the emission of the chemical by assuming that the chemical is released immediately. In addition, the model would assume that there is no air exchange with outdoor air or adjacent rooms. The air concentration in such a model is estimated as:

$$C = \frac{A}{V_{room}} \qquad \text{Eq. 1}$$

where:

- C = air concentration in the room,
- A = total amount of substance released, and
- V_{room} = room volume.

More complex model

Implementation of a more sophisticated description of the emission into this simple model and taking air exchange of the room with adjacent spaces and other sinks into account lead to a more realistic description of the modelled situation. Such a model requires solving a differential mass balance equation:

$$\frac{dC}{dt} = \frac{1}{V_{room}} \times \left\{ \sum_i S_i(t) - \sum_i \sigma_i(t) + \sum_j [C_j(t) - C(t)] \times Q_j \right\} \qquad \text{Eq. 2}$$

where:

- C = air concentration in the room
- V_{room} = room volume
- S_i = emission source i
- σ_i = sink i
- C_j = concentration in adjacent space j

> Q_j = air exchange rate with adjacent space j
>
> Increasing the model complexity in this manner, however, may introduce new and additional uncertainties into the exposure evaluation. More model parts and parameters have to be specified, but data of sufficient quality may not be available. Thus, making the model more complex and realistic need not lead to a decrease in the overall uncertainty of the exposure assessment.

As illustrated in the above example, equation 1 represents the simplest algorithm to express a room air concentration by dividing the amount by the room volume (EU, 2003). Equation 2 makes the model for estimating the room concentration more complex and time dependent. Equation 1 is used only for worst-case and low-tier assessments. Equation 2 is nearer to reality. If, however, the variables in the model are uncertain, total uncertainty of the results revealed by this model may be increased. These examples show that complexity of algorithms may introduce different qualitative and quantitative uncertainties into an assessment.

3.2.2.5 Extrapolation

The use of a model outside the domain for which it was developed may introduce an unknown level of uncertainty.

> **Example of extrapolation:**
>
> Using a model that was developed to estimate exposure to pesticides when spraying plants indoors to describe an outdoor situation will not correctly capture the different dispersion conditions outdoors.

3.2.2.6 Implementation of tools and software

Models implemented as software programs may suffer from errors in program code, hardware errors as well as differences in various computer operating systems.

> **Examples of tool and software implementation errors:**
>
> 1. Running a model by using Windows XP with settings specific for the United States versus Windows XP with German settings: A 70,00 kg (or 70 kg) body weight value (written in a very common European style) was read and calculated by one exposure model in the United States as 7000 kg, with similar errors in reading for other input parameters expressed with a decimal point.
> 2. Large spreadsheets with hundreds of dependencies might contain errors.

3.2.3 Parameter uncertainty

Exposure assessment involves the specification of values for parameters, either for direct determination of the exposure or as input for mechanistic or empirical or distribution-based models that are used to fill the exposure scenario with adequate information. Numerical values for exposure parameters are obtained using various approaches, such as the USEPA's Exposure Factors Handbook (USEPA, 1997a), the European Union's (EU) Technical Guidance Document (EU, 2003), the German XProb project (Mekel, 2003) and the European KTL's ExpoFacts (Vuori et al., 2006).

Sources of parameter uncertainty include the following:

- measurement errors (random or systematic);
- sample uncertainty;
- data type (e.g. surrogate data, expert judgement, default data, modelling data, measurement data);
- extrapolation uncertainty; and
- uncertainty in the determination of the statistical distribution used to represent distributed parameter values.

These sources of parameter uncertainty are described briefly below. Further details are given in section 5.1.

3.2.3.1 Measurement errors

Measurements of exposure parameters—for example, the indoor air concentrations of chemicals, time–activity patterns and the chemical composition of consumer products—will as a rule be subject to errors inherent in the methodology used, such as errors in the analytical methods used to measure chemical concentrations or inaccuracies in the survey data due to incorrect reporting by the participants. These errors may be categorized as random or systematic (biased) errors:

- *Random measurement errors*: These give rise to a variation around the "true" value: for instance, reading a scale with certain accuracy, reporting the use of a consumer product by a consumer with an equal chance of under- or over-reporting the actual use. Random measurement errors are often compounded with the true underlying variability in the quantity being measured (e.g. Zheng & Frey, 2005). For example, if one measures the ambient concentration of an air pollutant at a specific location, there is temporal variability in the true concentration. If the measurement method has a random component to the measurement error, then the variability in the measurements over time will be larger than the true variability in the ambient concentration. Failure to deconvolute random measurement error from the observed data can lead to an overestimate of variability.

Examples of random measurement errors:

1. Emond et al. (1997) showed that the method of sampling can significantly influence dust lead and children's blood lead levels. They showed, by field measurements of lead-contaminated

> dust using five dust lead measurement methods, variation over methods and surface types. Technician effects, inadvertent field exposure to lead, contamination of collection equipment and laboratory instrument error were found to contribute little to total measurement error.
> 2. The method chosen for studying nutrition habits may greatly influence estimations of exposure to food contaminants. Approaches to quantify consumption include:
>   (i) diet history protocol, where people are asked for their usual (e.g. over the last four weeks) foods consumed;
>   (ii) the 24-h recall, where people are asked what they ate the previous day;
>   (iii) real-time diaries, where people record what they eat (Willett, 1998); and
>   (iv) food frequency questionnaires, where people are asked a series of questions about how often they usually consumed a particular food in, for example, the past year or past month, as well as typical portion size.
>
> These diary studies may also include weighing of the food. The protocol period of these studies may vary from one day up to one week and may be repeated. All of these study designs have advantages and disadvantages, and their results have to be used according to the aim of the exposure assessment (e.g. whether a microbial outbreak or chronic exposure to heavy metals is being studied).

- *Systematic bias of measurements*: The average of the measurements of an exposure factor may differ from its "true" value. This difference is termed the bias and may be a result of, for example, incorrect calibration of the measuring apparatus or of over- or understating in questionnaires.

> **Example of systematic bias of measurements:**
>
> Taking nutrition survey data from a diet history study to assess the uptake of microbials from an outbreak will lead to systematic bias.

3.2.3.2 Sample uncertainty

Sample uncertainty is also referred to as statistical random sampling error. This type of uncertainty is often estimated assuming that data are sampled randomly and without replacement and that the data are random samples from an unknown population distribution. For example, when measuring body weights of different individuals, one might randomly sample a particular number of individuals and use the data to make an estimate of the interindividual variability in body weight for the entire population of similar individuals (e.g. for a similar age and sex cohort).

The first key requirement for making statistical inference from sample data is that it must be a representative sample. If the sample is not representative, then any statistic estimated from the sample can be biased. For example, if one wishes to know the breathing rate of 40- to 45-year-old adult males performing residential yard work, estimates based on data for other age groups or for other types of activities would not be representative.

If the sample is representative, then the second consideration is how artefacts of randomly choosing the samples lead to random variation in the estimate of statistics of interest, such as the mean or standard deviation of sample distribution of interindividual variability. While it is often assumed that a small sample of data is not or could not be representative, this is a common misconception. The issue of representativeness is one of study design and sampling strategy. If one has a representative sample, even if very small, then conventional statistical methods can be used to make inferences regarding sampling distributions of statistics, such as the mean. The implications of a small, random and representative sample are that the confidence intervals estimated for statistics of interest, such as the mean, can be very wide. The range of a confidence interval for a statistic is typically influenced by the sample size, the variability in the observed sample (i.e. the sample standard deviation) and which statistic is of interest. For example, the sampling distribution of a mean value is asymptotically normal as the sample size increases. However, the sampling distribution for the variance is positively skewed.

Examples of sample uncertainty:

1. A large sample of data (e.g. $n = 1000$) is obtained at random and represents a specific stratum of a population of interest, such as a specific age and sex cohort. The data represent observed interindividual variability (e.g. in body weight, in breathing rate). These data can be used to make a best estimate of the unknown population distribution, and conventional statistical methods can be used to infer confidence intervals regarding individual statistics (e.g. the mean) or for the entire observed distribution.
2. Similar to (1), but only a small sample (e.g. $n = 10$) is obtained. As long as the data are sampled randomly and are representative, the same statistical methods can be used. The key difference is that the estimated ranges of confidence intervals will be much wider.
3. A large sample of data is obtained, but the data are not random. They might be a convenience sample from people who self-select to participate in a voluntary study at a shopping centre. While such data can be stratified into cohort groups, it is possible that the study might have too large a representation of healthy persons or persons of higher socioeconomic status than the true population distribution for that cohort. As such, estimates of key exposure factors may be biased.
4. Similar to (3), but for a small sample of data. The fundamental problem of non-representativeness is the same, and inferences from these data are likely to provide biased estimates of exposure factors.
5. Extrapolating nutrition data from one country to another one, which is another example of non-representativeness.

3.2.3.3 Data type uncertainty

Data uncertainties depend on the type of data being used in the model, such as surrogate data, expert judgement, default data, modelled (extrapolated) data, etc.:

- *Surrogate data:* In the absence of situation-specific data, it is common that surrogate (or generic) data are used. Surrogate data are substitutes from one quantity that are used to estimate analogous or corresponding values of another quantity. If the surrogate data are not representative of the quantity of interest, then the use of surrogate data can potentially lead to biases in the mean estimate of the quantity of interest and can lead to mischaracterization of both interindividual variability and uncertainty.

Example of surrogate data:

The Technical Notes for Guidance on Human Exposure to Biocidal Products (EU, 2002a) provide indicative exposure values for a range of exposure scenarios (summarized in EU, 2002b). These have been derived from experiments and are suggested to be used in similar situations. Uncertainty is associated with the data selection procedure (i.e. the degree to which the selected data are representative for the situation that they are supposed to describe).

- *Professional (expert) judgement*: In situations where quantitative information on exposure factors is lacking, estimates of experts in the relevant field may be used. The process for eliciting expert judgement typically includes an expert selection procedure, expert elicitation protocol and reporting procedure. The expert selection procedure is typically intended to identify persons who have depth of domain knowledge in the topic area for which judgements are sought. The elicitation protocol is a formal procedure that involves a structured interview of an expert. The interview typically involves key steps, such as explaining why the elicitation is being done, structuring the elicitation to identify key parameters for which the expert is able to provide judgements, conditioning the expert to think about all relevant sources of uncertainty in the parameter, encoding the expert judgement using any of several accepted methods and validating the encoded judgement by checking for inconsistencies. The analyst might then use two or more judgements for the same parameter as input to an assessment, thus facing a decision of whether to produce exposure estimates based on each judgement separately or to combine them in some manner. Uncertainties can arise for several reasons. One is that the selected "experts" might not have been the most appropriate persons to select, in that they may not have adequate domain expertise. Another is that the selected experts may have motivational biases in that they feel obliged to defend previously stated positions, or they might want to influence the assessment results. The elicitation process itself must attempt to minimize or eliminate biases associated with cognitive heuristics that people use when constructing judgements regarding uncertainty. The analyst may fail to properly represent the range of expert judgement, depending on how judgements are used or combined in an assessment.

Example of expert judgement:

1. Nine experts were asked to rank substances (1–5 rankings) in a list according to their toxicological relevance. All rankings were presented (G. Heinemeyer, personal communication, 2005).
2. Multiple experts were asked to assess the uncertainty in concentration–response functions associated with human exposure to particulate matter. The experts were selected and their judgements encoded according to a formal protocol. The judgements of multiple experts were compared with each other and with available epidemiological data (Industrial Economics, Inc., 2004).

- *Default data*: Default values are reference values recommended for use for specific purposes—for instance, in screening-level assessments. The level of uncertainty associated with the use of default values (which may be distributions) depends on the procedure and the quality of the background data set used to derive them.

Example of default data:

Use of default parameters is one of the most frequently used approaches for exposure assessment where data are lacking and for low-tier estimations. Sometimes, worst-case values are used as model defaults to consider the conservative approach of the assessment, in accordance with values at level 1 of uncertainty, according to Paté-Cornell (1996b).

These data can be characterized as model variables/parameters that are thought to represent a conservative value at or above the upper range. However, they are not representative of a known range or distribution. Defaults are values that might not have been validated or evaluated, they

> need not reflect representativity and they do not meet other statistical criteria.
>
> Defaults for exposure assessment are given, for example, in the EU's Technical Guidance Document for new and existing chemicals (EU, 2003) (e.g. 0.01 cm as default for a fictive thickness of a layer of skin).
>
> Use of worst-case parameters is implying an unknown, but certainly high, degree of uncertainty in exposure assessments. Assessments that reveal risks by comparing exposure and hazard data should be repeated taking approaches considering more realistic models and parameters.

- *Extrapolated/modelled data*: Extrapolation is the inference of unknown data from known data (e.g. future data from past data) by analysing trends and making assumptions. Uncertainty is introduced by questions as to how representative the extrapolated data are for the situation in which they are used.

> **Examples of extrapolation uncertainty:**
>
> 1. The extrapolation of an estimation made for adults to children would imply a high degree of uncertainty. Children are not little adults. Normally, exposures are referred to body weight; however, the mechanisms that govern the physiological mechanisms for absorption, distribution and elimination (including metabolism) of substances in the body are linearly related not to body weight but to body surface (BgVV, 2001). Cohen Hubal et al. (2000) stated that data about children's exposures and activities are insufficient and that multimedia exposures to environmental contaminants cannot be assessed (see also IPCS, 2006a). In many assessments, defaults are taken, owing to a high degree of uncertainty in the assumptions and exposure estimates.
> 2. In the assessment of the uptake of a chemical after dermal exposure, for instance, the dermal permeability of the skin is often estimated using the Potts-Guy quantitative structure–activity relationship (Guy & Potts, 1992), which was derived from an experimental data set of in vitro measured steady-state skin permeations (Wilschut et al., 1995). Uncertainty in the use of a value for the skin permeation obtained this way comes from questions of how well a regression model based on K_{ow} and molecular weight predicts the skin permeability of a chemical that was not in the original data set, and how representative the steady-state permeability measured in vitro is for a (possibly) non-steady-state permeability in vivo (see also IPCS, 2006b).
> 3. A study designed for other purposes is used for exposure assessments (e.g. a food consumption survey performed for estimating "healthy nutrition" is used for estimating exposure to heavy metals).

3.2.3.5 Uncertainty in the determination of the statistical distribution used to represent distributed parameter values

Probability distribution models can be used to represent frequency distributions of variability or uncertainty distributions. When the data set represents variability for a model parameter, there can be uncertainty in any non-parametric statistic associated with the empirical data. For situations in which the data are a random, representative sample from an unbiased measurement or estimation technique, the uncertainty in a statistic could arise because of random sampling error (and thus be dependent on factors such as the sample size and range of variability within the data) and random measurement or estimation errors. The observed data can be corrected to remove the effect of known random measurement error to produce an "error-free" data set (Zheng & Frey, 2005).

If a parametric distribution (e.g. normal, lognormal, loglogistic) is fit to empirical data, then additional uncertainty can be introduced in the parameters of the fitted distribution. If the selected parametric distribution model is an appropriate representation of the data, then the uncertainty in the parameters of the fitted distribution will be based mainly, if not solely, on random sampling error associated primarily with the sample size and variance of the empirical data. Each parameter of the fitted distribution will have its own sampling distribution. Furthermore, any other statistical parameter of the fitted distribution, such as a particular percentile, will also have a sampling distribution. However, if the selected model is an inappropriate choice for representing the data set, then substantial biases in estimates of some statistics of the distribution, such as upper percentiles, must be considered.

For some empirical data sets for variability in a quantity, there can be one or more values that are either below a limit of detection of the measurement instrument or zero for structural reasons (e.g. zero consumption rate of a particular food by a particular person on a particular day). The former case is an example of missing data, whereas the latter is an example of a mixture distribution that is composed of one component that describes the frequency of zero values and a second component that might be a continuous distribution (e.g. consumption rates in this case).

For distributions that contain missing data, there are a variety of techniques that can be used, depending on the type of missingness. Perhaps the most common case of missing data is when one or more attempted measurements are below the detection limit, which are often referred to as "non-detects". This is referred to as a "left-censored" data set, in that small values below one or more threshold values (detection limits) are unobservable. Left-censored data are commonly dealt with using simplifying assumptions that, unfortunately, introduce bias into estimates of key statistics. For example, non-detects are often replaced with one half of the detection limit, and then mean values of the entire data set are estimated, taking into account both the non-detects and the detected values. For most data sets, the use of one half of the detection limit as a surrogate for the unknown non-detected value leads to a biased estimate of the mean of the empirical data set. Instead, statistical methods, such as maximum likelihood estimation, that use information regarding the proportion of the data set that is below one or more detection limits, the numerical values of the detection limits and the values of the observed data can provide more accurate estimates of a fitted distribution and its statistics (e.g. Zhao & Frey, 2004).

Structural uncertainties in a distribution can be represented by empirical distributions or a mixture of a discrete and parametric distribution, as described previously. Unless there is a need to partition the distribution into zero and non-zero components, failure to account for the frequency of zero values can lead to overestimation of the mean of the overall distribution.

> **Example of uncertainty in the choice of distribution for estimation of exposure to cadmium from iceberg lettuce consumption:**
>
> The estimated distributions of cadmium exposure from iceberg lettuce consumption and their statistics are displayed in Figure 3, using different distributions of cadmium concentration. For example, taking a lognormal distribution for simulation of the iceberg lettuce cadmium concentration, the 95th percentile was 18 ng/kg body weight per day, the normal distribution was

31 ng/kg body weight per day and the uniform distribution was 195 ng/kg body weight per day. Empirical data from the 1988–1989 German national nutrition survey were used to describe the iceberg lettuce consumption.

This example shows that the choice of distribution could make a large difference in the outcome of exposure assessment. Therefore, the data should be fitted against several distribution functions to get the best fit parameters to decrease uncertainty. Data collection and data generation therefore play dominant roles in probabilistic approaches. The probabilistic methodology convinces the assessors to use transparent data and shows the need to use sound statistical and survey methodology to get representative data.

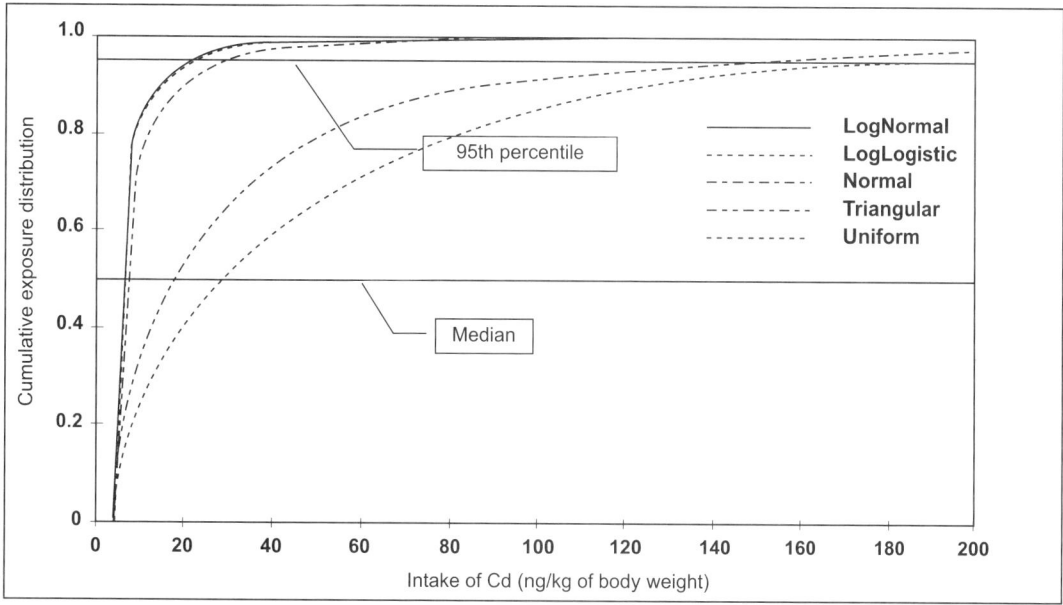

Figure 3: Distributions of cadmium intake (ng/kg body weight) from consumption of iceberg lettuce obtained using five different distribution functions of the cadmium concentrations. Contamination data are from the German "Lebensmittelmonitoring" programme (see BVL, 2006), and uptake data are from the 1988–1989 German national nutrition survey (Adolf et al., 1994).

4. TIERED APPROACH TO UNCERTAINTY ANALYSIS

Typically, exposure and risk assessments conducted during regulatory evaluations are performed in a tiered or phased approach. A tiered approach refers to a process in which the exposure or risk assessment progresses systematically from relatively simple to more complex. An important feature of a tiered analysis is that the exposure or risk assessment and the accompanying uncertainty analysis may be refined in successive iterations.

4.1 Regulatory background

Historically, much of the guidance for conducting environmental, exposure and risk assessments for air and multimedia pollutants has recommended considering a tiered or graded approach in regulatory impact and risk assessments. While the overarching consideration in conducting a tiered analysis is to increase the level of sophistication in the exposure, risk and uncertainty analysis when conducting a higher-tier analysis, the exact form of analysis in a given tier may vary depending on the specific technical and regulatory context. For instance, USEPA's Air Toxics Risk Assessment Technical Resource Manual (USEPA, 2004) advocates a three-tiered risk assessment process whereby each successive tier represents more complete characterization of variability and uncertainty as well as a corresponding increase in complexity and resource requirements. In this scheme, Tier 1 is represented as a relatively simple screening-level analysis using conservative and/or default exposure assumptions. Tier 2 analysis is represented as an intermediate-level analysis using more realistic exposure assumptions and more sophisticated qualitative or quantitative uncertainty analysis approaches. Tier 3 is represented as an advanced analysis using probabilistic exposure analysis techniques, such as the one- or two-dimensional Monte Carlo analysis methods, which incorporate full quantitative assessment of variability and uncertainty.

While Tier 1 analysis uses generic inputs, Tier 2 and Tier 3 analyses incorporate more site- or population-specific inputs in conducting the exposure and uncertainty analysis. A similar approach is also recommended by the USEPA in Volume III, Part A, of its Risk Assessment Guidance for Superfund (USEPA, 2001). In this guidance document, Tier 1 refers to conducting a point estimate risk assessment along with performing point estimate sensitivity analysis. Tier 2 analysis is characterized by conducting a one-dimensional Monte Carlo analysis along with probabilistic sensitivity analysis. USEPA (2001) assumes that a Tier 3 analysis involves the application of more advanced two-dimensional Monte Carlo simulations, microenvironmental exposure modelling or Bayesian methodologies, for separately characterizing variability and uncertainty in the predicted exposure or risk results. On the other hand, California's Office of Environmental Health Hazard Assessment advocates a four-tiered analysis under its "Hot Spots" air toxics programme (OEHHA, 2000). In this state programme in the United States, Tier 1 analysis refers to a point estimate method, whereas Tier 2 refers to a point estimate method using site-specific exposure parameters. A Tier 3 approach is characterized as a stochastic approach using exposure parameter distributions developed or endorsed by the Office of Environmental Health Hazard Assessment. A Tier 4 approach is considered a stochastic approach using site-specific distributions for the model inputs and parameters where defensible (OEHHA, 2000). A tiered approach is also recommended for exposure assessment in the "implementation projects" for the European chemicals regulation REACH, or the Registration, Evaluation, Authorisation and Restriction of Chemicals (EU, 2005), and for dietary exposure assessment by the European Food Safety Authority (EFSA, 2006). Tiered approaches to uncertainty are also used by other international organizations for non-exposure assessments, such as for contributions to global warming by the Intergovernmental Panel on Climate Change (IPCC, 2000).

4.2 Determination of the tiered level

Determination of an appropriate level of sophistication required from a particular uncertainty analysis depends on the intended purpose and scope of a given assessment. Most often tiered assessments are explicitly incorporated within regulatory and environmental risk management decision strategies. The level of detail in the quantification of assessment uncertainties, however, should match the degree of refinement in the underlying exposure or risk analysis. Where appropriate to an assessment objective, exposure assessments should be iteratively refined over time to incorporate new data, information and methods to reduce uncertainty and improve the characterization of variability. Lowest-tier analyses are often performed in screening-level regulatory and preliminary research applications. Intermediate-tier analyses are often considered during regulatory evaluations when screening-level analysis either indicates a level of potential concern or is not suited for the case at hand. The highest-tier analyses are often performed in response to regulatory compliance needs or for informing risk management decisions on suitable alternatives or trade-offs. Typically, higher-tier uncertainty analyses are based on more quantitative and comprehensive modelling of exposures or risks. The highest-tier analyses often provide a more quantitative evaluation of assessment uncertainties that also enables the regulators to determine how soon to act and whether to seek additional information on critical information or data gaps prior to reaching a decision.

The present monograph suggests a four-tier approach for characterizing the variability and/or uncertainty in the estimated exposure or risk results. These four tiers are described below.

4.2.1 Tier 0 (screening) uncertainty analysis

Tier 0 uncertainty analysis is performed for routine screening assessments, where it is not feasible to conduct a separate uncertainty characterization for each case. Instead, default uncertainty factors that have been established for the type of problem under consideration may be applied. These screening-level assessments are designed to demonstrate if the projected exposures or risks are unlikely to exceed reference values. Currently, most regulatory applications require, at the least, standardized or default methodologies for conducting exposure and risk assessments. These assessments also include often conservative defaults to reflect assessment uncertainties. These screening-level assessments are especially useful when it is not feasible to undertake more detailed sensitivity or uncertainty analyses (e.g. for performing high-throughput screening assessments). However, in conducting a Tier 0 uncertainty analysis, it is recommended that the default uncertainty factors should be derived from a more substantial (higher-tier) uncertainty analysis, in consultation with risk management, to ensure that the level of protection they afford is appropriate for the class of problems for which they are intended. Furthermore, it is suggested that within this exercise,

Tier 0 analysis may be done just once, but not repeated for every individual assessment. Even though Tier 0 assessments are practical to conduct, they are not suited for addressing problems that require a realistic identification of key factors and exposure conditions contributing to assessment outcomes and uncertainties. Higher-tier assessments are often needed to answer such questions.

> **Examples of Tier 0 analysis:**
>
> 1. A factor of 2–10 is often used as a default estimate of upper-bound uncertainties associated with ambient air quality modelling of exposures to particulates or gaseous pollutants.
> 2. The 1996 Food Quality Protection Act in the United States advocated the use of a 10-fold safety factor to address the special sensitivity of infants and young children to pesticides when a screening-level analysis of exposures is performed using the Standard Operating Procedures (SOPs) of the USEPA's Office of Pesticides.

4.2.2 Tier 1 (qualitative) uncertainty analysis

Where the screening assessment indicates a concern, a more case-specific uncertainty characterization is required to take account of any special circumstances of the case in hand (e.g. anything that might justify a smaller uncertainty factor than the default one) and to take account of any additional (higher-tier) data. Tier 1 analysis is intended to examine how likely it is that, and by how much, the exposure or risk levels of concern may be exceeded. Tier 1 is the simplest form of this enhanced uncertainty analysis, mostly based on a qualitative approach involving systematic identification and characterization of different sources of assessment uncertainties. The main objective of Tier 1 uncertainty analysis is to characterize the influence of each individual source of uncertainty independently on the results of the assessment. When the uncertainty analysis is qualitative in nature, the uncertainties in each of the major elements of the exposure or risk analysis are usually described, often together with a statement of the estimated magnitude and direction of the uncertainty. Moreover, to the extent possible, the combined effect of different sources of uncertainty on the exposure or risk predictions, perhaps based on a weight-of-evidence methodology in the absence of quantitative data, should also be considered. This might, in some cases, provide a sufficient basis to reach a risk management decision at Tier 1; if not, it would form the basis for performing Tier 2 uncertainty analysis.

> **Examples of Tier 1 uncertainty analysis:**
>
> 1. Examining the influence of the uncertainties in the key model variables (e.g. ranges of pollutant concentrations, differences in exposure durations, inhalation rates, body weights) that are used to predict high-end exposures of individuals.
> 2. Identifying the key sources of uncertainties in food consumption rates and dietary residue data during a dietary exposure and risk analysis, and subsequently examining their respective influence on model predictions.
> 3. Identifying and estimating the likely impact of key sources of uncertainties in conducting a residential pesticide exposure analysis (e.g. uncertainties associated with surface residue concentrations, frequency of hand contact with contaminated surfaces, pesticide transfer efficiency from different types of surfaces to the hand or body).

4.2.3 Tier 2 (deterministic) uncertainty analysis

In a higher-tier analysis, semiquantitative or quantitative sensitivity analysis, interval or perhaps factorial and probability-bound analyses are considered. The semiquantitative approach involves using available data to describe the potential range of values for the assessment parameters and performing sensitivity analysis to identify the parameters with the most impact on the exposure or risk predictions. Usually, Tier 2 uncertainty analysis consists of a deterministic point estimate sensitivity analysis. Sensitivity analysis in this context is often performed to identify the relative contribution of the uncertainty in a given parameter value (e.g. inhalation rate, emission rate) or a model component to the total uncertainty in the exposure or risk estimate. In a Tier 2 uncertainty analysis, the analysts usually examine the sensitivity of results to input assumptions by using modified input values. A sensitivity analysis thus performed may provide high, average or low predictions corresponding to the range of values considered for each of the inputs. Typically, these calculations are done for each variable at a time by holding the others constant, but they can also be done jointly by changing all of the inputs.

The results of the sensitivity analysis are typically presented as a percentage change in the baseline estimates corresponding to incremental change in the inputs to the exposure model. In some instances, when single-value high-end and central tendency point estimates do not provide sufficient information to the decision-makers, a qualitative uncertainty analysis can be conducted to determine the range of values within which the exposure or risk estimate is likely to fall and major factors that contribute to uncertainty (USEPA, 2004). The sensitivity analysis conducted provides a range of exposure or risk estimates that result from combinations of minimum and maximum values for some of the parameters and mid-range values for others (USEPA, 2004). Typically, a quantitative uncertainty analysis is implemented through probabilistic modelling and statistical analysis methods under the most advanced Tier 3 uncertainty analyses. The decision to proceed to this next tier depends mostly on the outcome of the Tier 2 analysis, but also on the regulatory requirements or research significance of the particular assessment.

> **Examples of Tier 2 uncertainty analysis:**
>
> 1. Deterministic sensitivity analysis performed during modelling of population exposures to ambient fine particulate matter by using high (H), medium (M) and low (L) values during the analysis of the impact of uncertainties associated with key inputs and parameters on model predictions (e.g. time spent outdoors [H = 95%, M = 80%, L = 50%], residential building infiltration fractions [H = 0.7, M = 0.5, L = 0.2], deposition rates [H = 0.4, M = 0.3, L = 0.1]).
> 2. Deterministic sensitivity analysis conducted using SOP algorithms for estimating children's exposures to residential use pesticides, in which in addition to the SOP defaults, upper- and lower-bound estimates are used for each of the exposure variables (e.g. for hand-to-mouth contact frequencies, amount of pesticides applied to surfaces, pesticide residue transfer coefficients) in the calculation of combined exposure uncertainties.

4.2.4 Tier 3 (probabilistic) uncertainty analysis

Tier 3 analyses rely upon probabilistic methods to characterize the individual and combined effects of input and parameter uncertainties on the predicted results. Moreover, in some Tier 3 analyses, separate contributions of variability and uncertainty to overall assessment uncertainties may be differentiated. The starting point for any Tier 3 analysis is the quantification of probability distributions for each of the key exposure or risk model input values (e.g. mean and standard deviation of fitted statistical distributions, such as normal or lognormal distributions). These are often derived from existing measured or modelled values and in some cases based on expert judgements. Tier 3 uncertainty analysis examines the combined influence of the input uncertainties on the predictions by propagating either analytically (e.g. Taylor series approximation) or numerically (e.g. Monte Carlo simulation) parameter and input value uncertainties, as appropriate. When few parameters are involved in the exposure calculations, analytical methods may be in order. However, more complex model formulations often dictate the need for using numerical (e.g. Monte Carlo, Bayesian) techniques for sensitivity and uncertainty analysis. Most Tier 3 uncertainty analyses do not differentiate variability from uncertainty (e.g. with one-dimensional Monte Carlo analysis). Consequently, in such instances, it is not possible to readily distinguish the relative contribution of inherent variability in the exposure or risk factors from knowledge-based uncertainties to total assessment uncertainties.

More comprehensive quantitative analyses of exposure assessment uncertainties often rely upon modelling approaches that separately characterize variability and uncertainty in the model inputs and parameters. Examples include two-dimensional Monte Carlo analysis, microenvironmental exposure modelling, geostatistical analysis of concentrations and exposure factors and Bayesian statistics. It is important to note that the interpretation of results from one-dimensional Monte Carlo analysis can be different from that derived from two-dimensional Monte Carlo analysis. For example, the distribution of values predicted by a one-dimensional Monte Carlo analysis (typically plotted as a cumulative distribution function) usually represents the uncertainty distribution for a randomly drawn individual from the study population, whereas the variability distribution generated from the first stage of a two-dimensional Monte Carlo model represents the variability in the predicted median exposures. Methods used to characterize uncertainty in the inputs or parameters of the exposure models are based on fitting either parametric probability distributions or non-parametric probability distributions for the key variables selected for uncertainty characterization. Tier 3 probabilistic analyses also consider moderate or strong correlations or dependencies that exist between the model input variables. However, quite often not all the model variables are considered in a formal uncertainty analysis. For instance, human exposure model inputs that are based on survey data (e.g. time–activity data, dietary food consumption data) are often used in predicting only the inherent variability in exposures of individuals within the study population.

> **Principle 4**
>
> *The presence or absence of moderate to strong dependencies between model inputs is to be discussed and appropriately accounted for in the analysis.*

In principle, the outputs from variability and uncertainty analysis are used to quantify the nature of the variability in the predicted distribution of the exposures and the uncertainties associated with different percentiles of the predicted population exposure or risk estimates. The combined sensitivity and uncertainty are also used in a two-dimensional probabilistic exposure or dose assessment, in order to determine either the uncertainty about exposure (or dose) at a given percentile or the uncertainty about percentile for a given exposure (or dose) level. In addition, uncertainty analysis based on multivariate correlation and regression techniques shows the relative contribution of each input to the overall analysis variance. These results are quite informative for risk managers in identifying key factors influencing exposures and risks to different segments of the population (e.g. the entire population or the potentially highly exposed, such as those above the predicted 90th percentile exposures). This type of detailed information is also valuable for targeting future data collection activities on those information elements that have been determined to contribute most to the overall uncertainty in the exposure or risk results. Examples of output from a two-dimensional probabilistic exposure and dose modelling application for a recent wood treatment case-study for children's potential exposure to arsenic, using the USEPA's SHEDS (Stochastic Human Exposure and Dose Simulation) model (Zartarian et al., 2006), are shown in Figures 4 and 5.

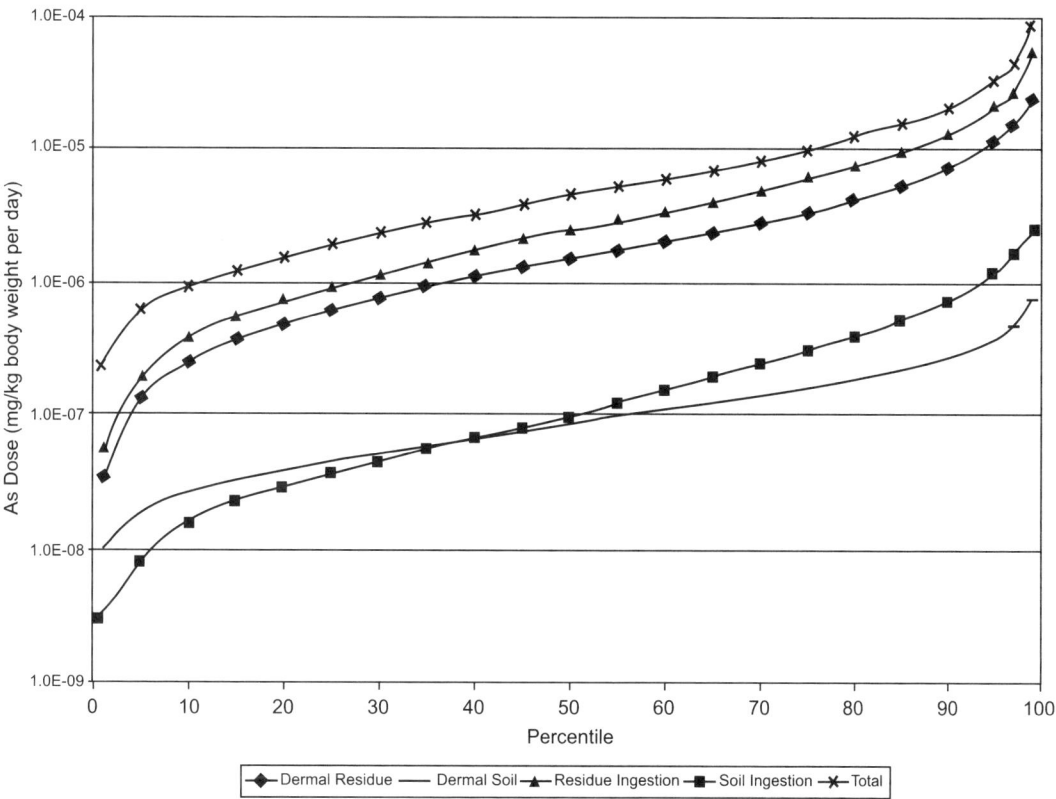

Figure 4: Relative contribution by exposure route to predicted dose: Estimated population lifetime average daily dose of arsenic for children exposed to chromated copper arsenate (CCA)-treated wood playsets and decks in warm climate regions (from Zartarian et al., 2006).

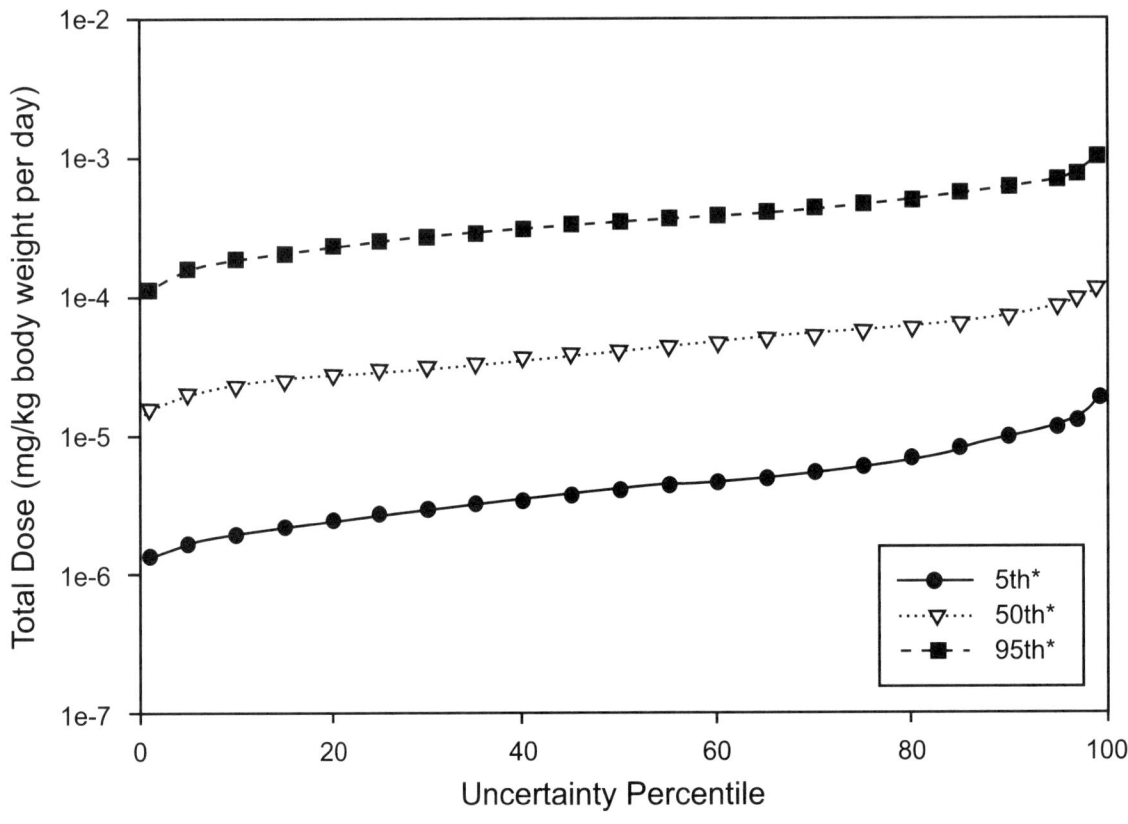

* 5th, 50th, and 95th percentiles from each simulation.

Figure 5: Predicted uncertainty cumulative distribution functions associated with three selected variability percentiles of the estimated annual average daily dose distributions for arsenic exposures from contact with CCA-treated wood playsets and decks in warm climate regions (from Xue et al., 2006).

Examples of Tier 3 uncertainty analysis:

1. Using a one-dimensional Monte Carlo analysis to estimate population exposure and dose uncertainty distributions for particulate matter, where model inputs and parameters (e.g. ambient concentrations, indoor particulate matter emission rates from environmental tobacco smoke, indoor air exchange rates, building penetration values, particle deposition rates) are represented probabilistically with distributions statistically fitted to all available relevant data.
2. Conducting a two-dimensional Monte Carlo modelling analysis for exposures to particulate matter, air toxics, pesticides or metals, in which both variability and uncertainty in model inputs and parameters are separately quantified explicitly, and their individual as well as their combined effects on model results are estimated using either parametric or non-parametric sensitivity analysis techniques (Burke et al., 2001; Zartarian et al., 2005, 2006; Xue et al., 2006).

4.3 Summary of the tiered approach

The amount of effort and detail devoted to analysing uncertainties should be proportionate to the needs of the problem, and so a tiered approach is recommended.

Part 1: Guidance Document on Characterizing and Communicating Uncertainty in Exposure Assessment

Tier 0 exposure assessments, which are commonly used for first-tier screening purposes, do not require an analysis of uncertainty on every occasion, provided they include appropriate conservative assumptions or safety factors to take account of uncertainty.

Higher-tier assessments do not require the quantification of every uncertainty. Therefore, a tiered approach is proposed where each individual source of uncertainty in an assessment may be treated at one of three tiers, beginning with qualitative approaches (Tier 1) and progressing to deterministic (Tier 2) or probabilistic approaches (Tier 3) when appropriate. Within a single uncertainty assessment, different sources of uncertainty may be treated at different tiers. Higher-tier methods are targeted on those uncertainties that have most influence on the assessment outcome. It is never practical to treat all uncertainties probabilistically; therefore, even in a very refined assessment, some uncertainties will still be treated at the lower tiers.

Example of the tiered approach to uncertainty analysis:

Within a single assessment, different sources of uncertainty may be treated at different tiers. For example, in an assessment of dietary exposure to a chemical, a screening assessment might use default values (Tier 0) for body weight and food consumption, combined with a conservative deterministic value (Tier 2) for concentration of the chemical in food (e.g. the highest measured value). The resulting exposure estimate might be accompanied by a qualitative evaluation (Tier 1) of uncertainties affecting the concentration data (e.g. the degree of measurement and sampling uncertainty). If a higher-tier assessment were required, various options for refinement could be considered, including, for example, the following:

- the default values for body weight and food consumption might be replaced with deterministic values (Tier 2) for a representative sample of consumers, obtained from a dietary survey; and
- probabilistic methods (Tier 3) might be used to provide a quantitative estimate of measurement and sampling uncertainty in the concentration data.

In the final assessment, some uncertainties may be quantified deterministically (Tier 2) or probabilistically (Tier 3). Sources of uncertainty that remain unquantified should be evaluated qualitatively (Tier 1). The overall assessment might be described as Tier 3 (because some sources of uncertainty are treated probabilistically), but it also contains elements at Tiers 1 and 2.

5. UNCERTAINTY CHARACTERIZATION METHODS, INTERPRETATION AND USE

In this chapter, both qualitative and quantitative approaches for characterizing uncertainty are described. We illustrate how these approaches apply and provide insight on the different tiers of an uncertainty analysis.

5.1 Qualitative uncertainty characterization

5.1.1 Rationale and objective

Currently, there are inconsistencies in the application and methodology for uncertainty analysis in exposure assessment. While several sophisticated quantitative techniques exist, their general application is hampered not only by their complexity (and resulting need for considerable supporting information) but also by the lack of methodology to facilitate the specification of uncertainty sources prior to the quantification of their specific weight.

Depending on the purpose of an assessment (e.g. screening to designate non-priorities for further action) or the availability of relevant data, it is not always possible or necessary to conduct quantitative uncertainty analysis in exposure assessment. In contrast, systematic qualitative characterization of the sources of uncertainty is encouraged, as it provides the appropriate degree of confidence in outcome and associated recommendations balanced by the identification of critical data gaps. It permits optimum use of (often) limited data in specific circumstances, with a clear delineation of relative uncertainty to indicate choices relevant to data generation and/or decision-making.

In view of the often considerable limitations of available data supporting exposure assessment, which sometimes limit the extent of uncertainty quantification and the need to explicitly identify sources of uncertainty prior to their quantification, this section provides an overview of existing concepts and proposes a harmonized approach for the qualitative analysis of uncertainty in exposure assessment.

The objective of qualitative characterization of uncertainty includes transparency in identifying key sources of uncertainty as an aid to risk managers who may need to make decisions in the absence of extensive data sets for substances with limited information—a prerequisite to quantification of uncertainty for substances with more extensive data.

The aim of qualitative characterization of uncertainty is to provide a conceptual basis for the systematic assessment of uncertainty in decision support processes such as exposure assessment. It focuses on uncertainty perceived from the point of view of assessors providing information to support policy decisions—that is, uncertainty regarding the analytical outcomes and conclusions of the exposure assessment.

The inclusive description of the components mentioned below is offered in the context of increasing transparency, although the limitations of available data may preclude consideration of all aspects. In all cases, the objective is to identify the principal sources of uncertainty that are influential in determining the outcome of the assessment and next steps, rather than simply listing unweighted gaps in information. Depending on the nature of information available, the reader is also referred to alternative, potentially simpler approaches to qualification of uncertainties, such as that presented in section 4.2.1 of EFSA (2006).

5.1.2 Methodology for qualitative uncertainty characterization

The methodology for qualitatively characterizing the uncertainty of the exposure assessment consists of two basic steps:

1) specification of uncertainty sources; and
2) qualitative characterization of uncertainty.

These steps are analysed in the sections that follow.

5.1.2.1 Specification of the sources of uncertainty

The three main classes of sources of uncertainty (section 3.2) are "scenario uncertainty", "model uncertainty" (in both conceptual model formulation and mathematical model formulation) and "parameter uncertainty" (both epistemic and aleatory). The uncertainty of the "conceptual model" source concentrates on the relationship between the selected model and the scenario under consideration.

The nature and extent of the qualitative characterization of these sources of uncertainty are necessarily dependent on the objective of the exposure assessment and the appropriate form of output for its intended purpose. Prior to initiating the development of any assessment, its intended purpose must be clearly articulated.

Each of the three basic sources of uncertainty—"scenario", "model" and "parameter"—can be further detailed in order to characterize each basic component separately (Table 1).

Table 1: Detailed sources of uncertainty.

Basic source of uncertainty	Detailed sources of uncertainty
Scenario	Agent
	Exposed population
	Microenvironment
	Spatial and temporal information
	Population activity
	Risk management measure
	Exposure pathway
	Exposure event
	Exposure route

Basic source of uncertainty	Detailed sources of uncertainty
Model	Model assumption
	Model dependency
	Model structure
	Equation
	Model extrapolation
	Model implementation
Parameter	Data source
	Data dependency
	Data value
	Data unit

Principle 5

Data, expert judgement or both should be used to inform the specification of uncertainties for scenarios, models and model parameters.

5.1.2.2 Qualitative characterization of uncertainty

Components of the qualitative characterization of uncertainty are listed below (see also Figure 6):

1) qualitatively evaluate the *level of uncertainty* of each specified source;
2) define the major sources of uncertainty;
3) qualitatively evaluate the *appraisal of the knowledge base* of each major source;
4) determine the controversial sources of uncertainty;
5) qualitatively evaluate the *subjectivity of choices* of each controversial source; and
6) reiterate this methodology until the output satisfies stakeholders.

The extent to which each item is taken into consideration is a function of the nature of the relevant database and the purpose of the exposure assessment. The objective is to identify the sources of uncertainty that are most influential in determining the outcome of an exposure assessment.

The level of sophistication with which uncertainty is assessed is necessarily dependent on the use that will be made of the information (Paté-Cornell, 1996a). Sometimes, a "level zero" analysis of uncertainty is all that is needed, simply asking: are there any major sources of uncertainty? At a slightly higher level, we can ask: what are the controversial sources of uncertainty? If we believe that we can afford to incur this uncertainty, the analysis can end there.

The three "three-dimensional" qualitative evaluation steps and their application in the overall qualitative evaluation process are detailed below.

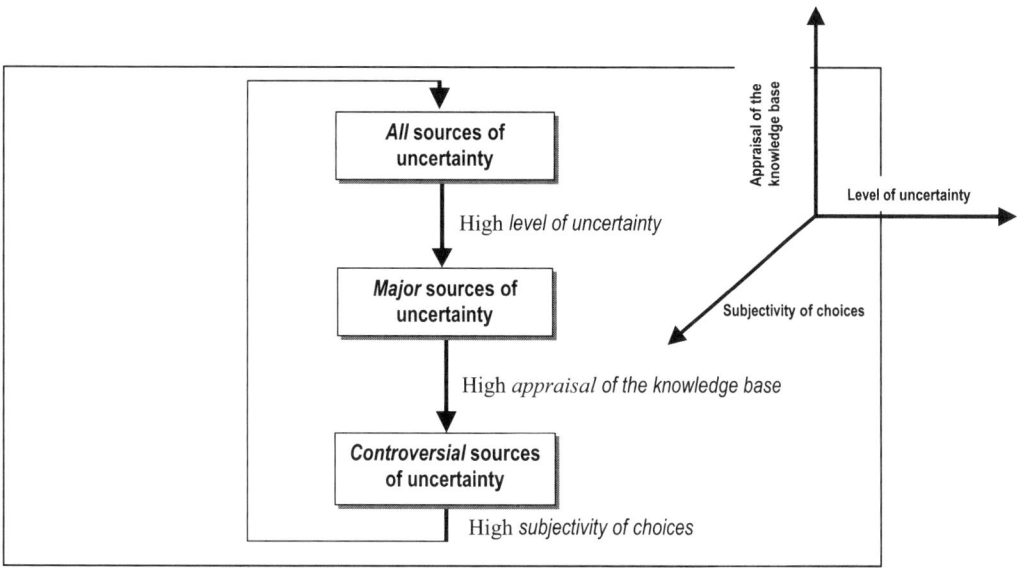

Figure 6: Reduction of the number of sources of uncertainty through the three-dimensional characteristics of uncertainty (see inset): level of uncertainty, appraisal of the knowledge base and subjectivity of choices

1) Level of uncertainty

The "level of uncertainty" is essentially an expression of the *degree of severity of the uncertainty*, seen from the assessors' perspective.

A scale ranging from "low" to "high" can be used to assess the sensitivity of the exposure assessment outputs to changes in the other sources being specified, as illustrated in Figure 7.

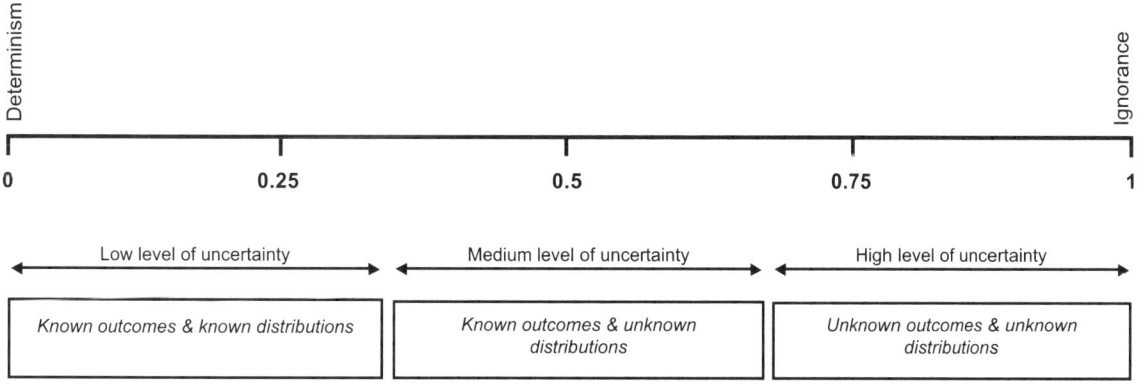

Figure 7: The scale of level of uncertainty (adapted from Walker et al., 2003; Krayer von Krauss & Janssen, 2005)

A "low" level on the scale implies that a large change in the source would have only a small effect on the results, a "medium" level implies that a change would have a proportional effect and a "high" level implies that a small change would have a large effect.

The most obvious example of a low level of uncertainty is the measurement uncertainty associated with parameters. Measurement uncertainty stems from the fact that measurement can practically never precisely represent the "true" value of that which is being measured. Uncertainty due to ignorance can be further divided into *reducible ignorance* and *irreducible ignorance*. Reducible ignorance may be resolved by conducting further research, which implies that it might be possible to achieve a better understanding. Irreducible ignorance applies when neither research nor development can provide sufficient knowledge about the essential relationships. Irreducible ignorance is also called *indeterminacy* (Walker et al., 2003).

2) Appraisal of the knowledge base

"Appraisal of the knowledge base" focuses on the adequacy of the available knowledge base for the exposure assessment (e.g. identification of data gaps and their impact on outcome). It involves questions such as: What criteria to evaluate quality are relevant for answering the assessment questions? What knowledge and methods are needed to obtain answers of the required quality? In the light of existing controversies and weaknesses in the knowledge base, what are the most significant bottlenecks? What effect do these bottlenecks have on the quality of the results, and what actions should be taken to clear them?

Examples of criteria for evaluating the uncertainty of the knowledge base are accuracy, reliability, plausibility, scientific consistency and robustness. These criteria are detailed in Table 2.

Table 2: Detailed specification of each criterion evaluating the knowledge base uncertainty.

	Appraisal of the knowledge base
Criteria	**Approaches and considerations**
Accuracy	1) establishing the knowledge base needed to obtain answers of the required quality
	2) signalling controversies with respect to the knowledge base
	3) identifying the most important bottlenecks in the available knowledge
	4) determining the impact of these bottlenecks on the quality of the results
	5) assessing the assumptions covering the knowledge gaps
Reliability	1) criticizing the knowledge base severely on factual and methodological grounds
	2) identifying the scientific status of the knowledge base
	3) determining the quality soundness of the knowledge base
	4) assessing the appropriateness of judgemental estimates of level of confidence

Part 1: Guidance Document on Characterizing and Communicating Uncertainty in Exposure Assessment

	Appraisal of the knowledge base
Criteria	**Approaches and considerations**
Plausibility	1) determining the completeness of the knowledge base
	2) acknowledging ignorance when applicable
	3) analysing the possibility of changes in underlying processes over time
	4) considering well established observations
Scientific consistency	1) assessing the consistency of scientific support
	2) assessing the maturity of the underlying science
	3) assessing the scientific limitations
	4) analysing the degree to which understanding is based on fundamental concepts tested in other areas
Robustness	1) assessing the predictability of the values and of the results
	2) assessing the dependency relationships

A scale ranging from "low" to "high" can be used to evaluate the uncertainty of the knowledge base, as illustrated in Figure 8.

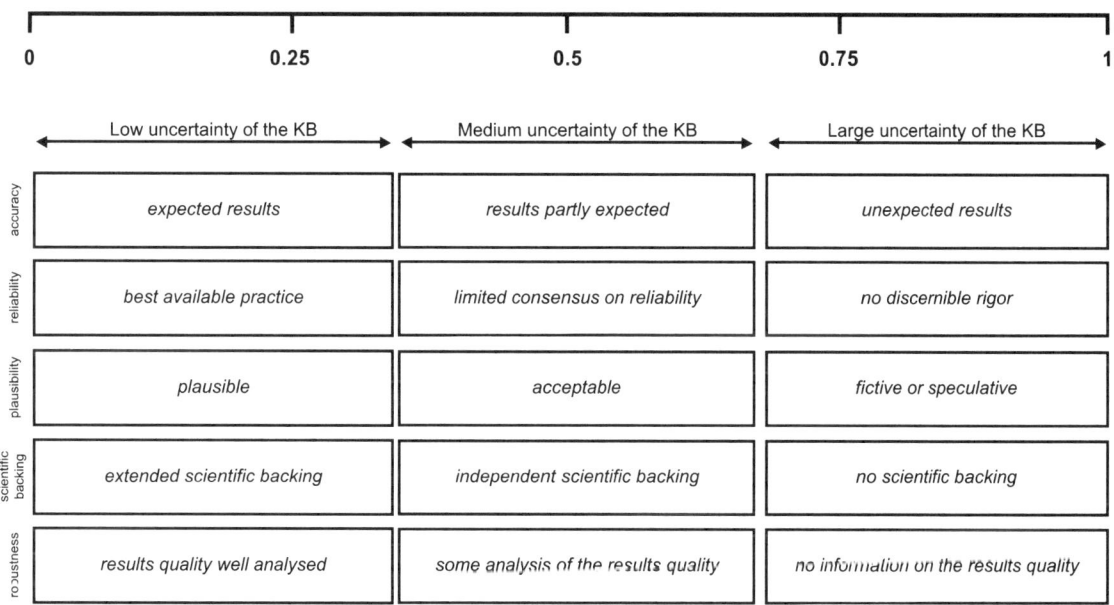

Figure 8: The scale of knowledge base (KB) uncertainty (adapted from van der Sluijs et al., 2005)

3) Subjectivity of choices

"Subjectivity of choices" delivers insight into the choice processes of the exposure assessors when they have made assumptions during the exposure assessment and particularly focuses on the value-ladenness of assumptions, starting from the viewpoint of the exposure assessors carrying out the assessment.

Examples of criteria for evaluating the subjectivity of choices are choice space, intersubjectivity among peers and among stakeholders, influence of situational limitations (e.g. money, tools and time) on choices, sensitivity of choices to the analysts' interests and influence of choices on results. These criteria are detailed in Table 3.

Table 3: Detailed specification of each criterion evaluating the uncertainty related to the subjectivity of choices.

Subjectivity of choices	
Criteria	*Approaches and considerations*
Choice space	1. spanning alternative choices
Intersubjectivity among peers and among stakeholders	2. specifying the similarity of choices among peers and among stakeholders
	3. specifying the controversy of choices among peers and among stakeholders
Influence of situational limitations (e.g. money, tools and time) on choices	4. determining the influence of situational limitations on the choices
Sensitivity of choices to the analysts' interests	5. assessing the sensitivity of the choices to the analysts' interests
Influence of choices on results	6. determining the influence of the choices on the results

A scale ranging from "low" to "high" can be used to evaluate the uncertainty of the subjectivity of choices, as illustrated in Figure 9.

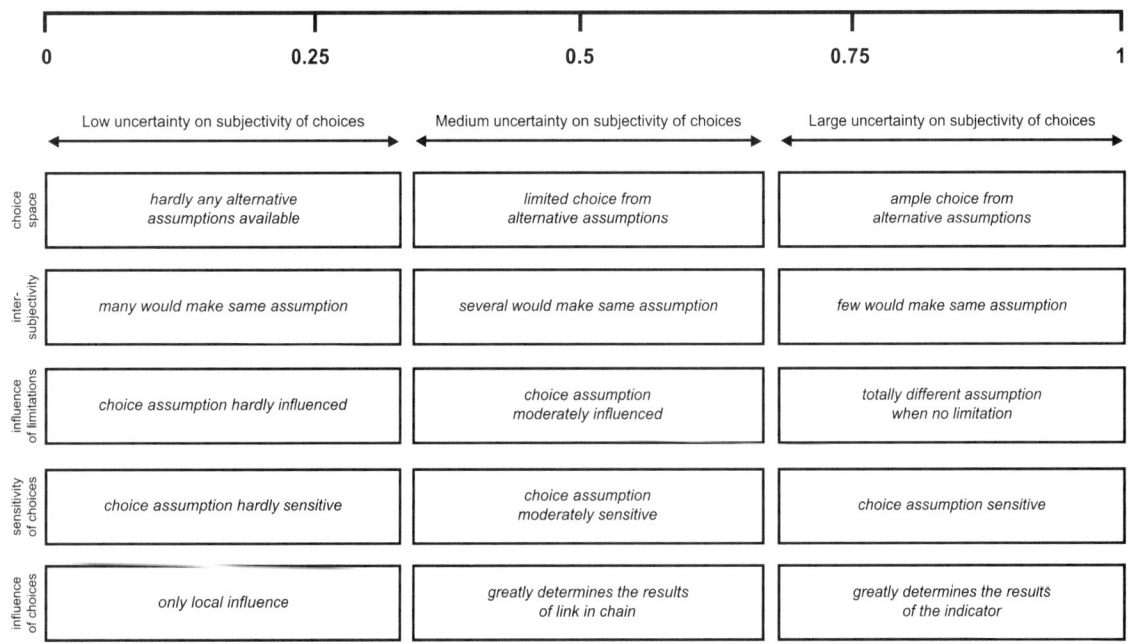

Figure 9: The scale of uncertainty related to subjectivity of choices (adapted from van der Sluijs et al., 2005)

4) Qualitative evaluation of the uncertainty

Each identified source of uncertainty is evaluated against the selected characteristic of uncertainty (i.e. not applicable or low, medium or high), which leads to a map of qualitative values.

In a first step, both exposure assessors and risk managers should give a qualitative indication of the *level of uncertainty* of each source and the way in which this uncertainty could influence the final output of the exposure assessment.

In a second step, both exposure assessors and risk managers should look closely at the *appraisal of knowledge base* to see what the reasons for the recognized levels of uncertainty are and what actions (such as research) can be discerned to deal effectively with that uncertainty in order to make the assessment more robust.

In a final step, both exposure assessors and risk managers and eventually the involved stakeholders should understand the range of factors influencing the *subjectivity of choices* and assumptions of exposure assessors.

It is essential to provide risk managers with an assessment of the overall degree of uncertainty in the assessment outcome. This should integrate all three dimensions of uncertainty, from all parts of the assessment. Integration of qualitative uncertainties is inevitably subjective, so it is important to document the reasoning so that others can evaluate the conclusions that are reached.

The transparency of qualitative evaluation of uncertainty may be enhanced through the use of an evaluation matrix (Table 4), where the considered *sources* of uncertainty are listed in lines and the *characteristics* of uncertainty (i.e. qualitative extent of the uncertainty) in columns, together with their justification. Included in a cell at the intersection of a source and characteristic is an evaluation of "not applicable", "low", "medium" or "high", according to the considered uncertainty characteristic for the source. The use of common descriptors in an evaluation matrix of this nature could lead to greater convergence in transparency by avoiding the use of inconsistent or uncritical terminology for uncertainty often included in exposure assessments.

Table 4: Qualitative evaluation matrix for exposure assessment.

Qualitative evaluation of the uncertainty	*Qualitative characterization of uncertainty*	
	Characteristic of uncertainty	***Justification***
Sources of uncertainty $source_k$	<value ∈ {NA, Low, Medium, High}> where NA stands for not applicable	<free textual field>

Thus, each exposure assessment has one or more qualitative evaluation matrices depending on the selected characteristics of uncertainty.

Annex 1 provides a case-study of a qualitative characterization of uncertainties in an exposure assessment. Table A1.2 in Annex 1 details the evaluation throughout the three-dimensional characteristics. Included is an overall conclusion on sensitivity—that is, those aspects that have the most significant impact on the outcome of the assessment, as better data collected on these features would considerably reduce the measure of uncertainty. An example of the overall conclusion is given in section A1.5 of Annex 1. The main uncertainties identified in the assessment are tabulated, as illustrated in Table 5, and a brief explanation of the weights given to them in reaching an overall conclusion is provided. In addition, a textual description of the qualitative characterization of tabular output should include an indication of overall uncertainty, based on the collective impact of each of the sources.

Table 5: Example of tabular approach to summarizing the main uncertainties affecting an assessment.

Sources of uncertainty	*Characteristics of uncertainty*		
	Level of uncertainty	Appraisal of knowledge base	Subjectivity of choices
Scenario	High		Medium
Model: Conceptual	Medium		
Model: Mathematical	High	Low	
Parameters	High		

5.1.3 Conclusion

Through the review of approaches to explicit qualitative consideration of contributing sources, this section offers a framework to facilitate and promote a qualitative consideration of the impact of uncertainties on exposure assessment where data are very limited and/or as a prelude to more quantitative characterization of uncertainties. Transparency to address uncertainties and specification of those uncertainties that impact most on outcome are essential to effective decision-making in risk management.

5.2 Quantitative uncertainty characterization

This section provides an overview of common methods for quantitative uncertainty analysis of inputs to models and the associated impact on model outputs. Furthermore, consideration is given to methods for analysis of both variability and uncertainty. In practice, commonly used methods for quantification of variability, uncertainty or both are typically based on numerical simulation methods, such as Monte Carlo simulation or Latin hypercube sampling. However, there are other techniques that can be applied to the analysis of uncertainty, some of which are non-probabilistic. Examples of these are interval analysis and fuzzy methods. The latter are briefly reviewed. Since probabilistic methods are commonly used in practice, these methods receive more detailed treatment here. The use of quantitative methods for variability and uncertainty is consistent with, or informed by, the key hallmarks of data quality, such as appropriateness, transparency, accuracy and integrity, as described in Part 2 of this Harmonization Project Document.

Although the focus here is on quantifying variability and uncertainty in model inputs and assessing their effect on model outputs, uncertainties in scenarios and models are also important. As yet, there appears to be no formalized methodology for dealing quantitatively with uncertainty in scenarios. Scenario uncertainty is typically associated with qualitative issues regarding what is included or excluded and is dependent on the state of knowledge regarding the real-world system and judgement regarding which aspects of the real-world system are salient with respect to human exposures. Decisions regarding what to include or exclude from a scenario could be recast as hypotheses regarding which agents, pathways, microenvironments and so on contribute significantly to the overall exposure of interest. Thus, decisions whether to include or exclude a particular aspect of a scenario could be subject to scientific methods. In practice, however, the use of qualitative methods tends to be more common, given the absence of a formal quantitative methodology.

Structural uncertainties in models can be dealt with in a variety of ways, including (1) parameterization of a general model that can be reduced to alternative functional forms (e.g. Morgan & Henrion, 1990), (2) enumeration of alternative models in a probability tree (e.g. Evans et al., 1994), (3) assessment of critical assumptions within a model, (4) assessment of the pedigree of a model and (5) assessment of model quality. The first two of these are quantitative methods, whereas the others are qualitative. In practice, a typical approach is to compare estimates made separately with two or more models. However, the models may not be independent of each other with respect to their basis in theory or data. Thus, an apparently favourable comparison of models may indicate only consistency, rather than accuracy.

5.2.1 Intervals and probability bounds

Ferson (1996) points out that there is a class of problems in which information may be known regarding upper and lower bounds for a particular variable, but not regarding a probability distribution. The model output in such cases is an interval, rather than a distribution. Such problems are more appropriately dealt with using interval methods rather than imposing probabilistic assumptions upon each input. Interval methods can be extended to situations in which marginal probability distributions are specified for each model input but for which the dependence between the distributions is not known. Thus, rather than assume statistical independence, or any particular correlation or more complex form of dependency, a bounding technique can be used to specify the range within which the model output distribution must be bounded.

Some would argue that if there is sufficient information upon which to quantify ranges, then there is also likely information upon which to base a judgement regarding the type of distribution that could be used to describe uncertainty in the input. Interval methods, however, may be useful for problems in which there may be complex dependencies between inputs but for which the dependencies are not known. A disadvantage of interval methods is that the predicted intervals for a model output can be quite wide, since they are informed only by the end-points of the ranges for each input. Interval methods can be useful as a quality assurance check on the results of a Monte Carlo simulation or other method, since the results from other methods should be enclosed by the results from the interval method.

As a simple illustration of interval methods, consider the example given by Ferson (1996) pertaining to multiplication of two inputs. Input A has an interval of [0.2, 0.4], and Input B has an interval of [0.3, 0.5]. The interval for the model output is [0.06, 0.2]. The output interval is the narrowest possible interval that accounts for all possible forms of dependence between A and B.

Many analysts are tempted to assign a uniform distribution when only a minimum value and a maximum value are specified for an input. Such an assignment is justified on the theoretical basis of maximum entropy. However, it is clear that assuming a probability distribution within the specified range involves presuming more information than simply assigning an interval. Furthermore, if inputs A and B are each assigned distributions, then there is the question of whether the two inputs are statistically independent. Each of these assumptions implies more information on the part of experts or the analyst. Ferson (1996) argues that if such information is not available, then there is not justification for making such assumptions simply because they are convenient. Of course, in many cases, the state of knowledge may adequately support judgements regarding the probability distribution for each input and the nature of the dependence, if any, between them.

A variation on the use of intervals is the use of discretized strata to represent a continuous distribution. For example, as described in section A2.2.4 of Annex 2, the "factorial design" method involves representing inputs to a model as nominal values that are described as low, medium and high. The numerical estimates associated with these ranges could be the minimum, median and maximum values from the corresponding continuous distribution. A similar but more formal method, known as *discrete probability distribution* (DPD) arithmetic, involves representing a continuous distribution as a discrete distribution, also with low, medium and high ranges. However, the numerical values of a DPD for each of these three ranges should be the mean of each range, in order to more accurately approximate the mean and central moments of the original continuous distribution.

5.2.2 Fuzzy methods

Fuzzy methods were introduced to represent and manipulate data and information possessing no statistical uncertainties (Zadeh, 1965). Fuzzy methods differ from statistical methods in that they do not conform to axioms of probability. Fuzzy methods are based upon fuzzy sets (e.g. Jablonowski, 1998). An element of a fuzzy set, such as a particular number for an input to a model, has a grade of membership in the set. The grade of membership is different in concept from probability and is often referred to simply as "membership". Membership is a quantitative noncommittal measure of imperfect knowledge. For example, suppose that the height of a person is classified as "tall" or "not tall". In a fuzzy representation, the person's height might be given a partial membership of, say, 0.7 in the tall set and therefore would have a partial membership of 0.3 in the "not tall" set.

Fuzzy methods are suitable for approximate reasoning (Isukapalli & Georgopoulos, 2001), especially for analysis of systems where uncertainty arises due to vagueness or "fuzziness" or incomplete information rather than due to randomness alone (Evans et al., 1986). The advantage of these methods is that they can characterize non-random uncertainties arising from vagueness or incomplete information and give an approximate estimate of the uncertainties. The limitations of the fuzzy methods are that (1) they cannot provide a precise estimate of uncertainty, but only an approximate estimation, and (2) they might not work for situations involving uncertainty arising from random sampling error.

5.2.3 Probabilistic methods

Probabilistic methods for quantification of variability and uncertainty are used in practice to estimate the exposures for different percentiles of exposed populations and to estimate the precision of the exposure estimates for any given percentile. These methods are quantitative. As indicated in section 1.6, probabilistic methods can be applied to quantify variability only, uncertainty only, variability and uncertainty co-mingled or variability and uncertainty that are distinguished. The first three are accomplished using "one-dimensional" analysis, whereas the latter is accomplished using "two-dimensional" approaches. For a one-dimensional analysis, there is a unique value of any given variable associated with a percentile of the distribution. For example, there is a unique estimate of exposure at the 95th percentile of the distribution of interindividual variability in exposure. For a two-dimensional analysis, for any given level of exposure, there is a distribution regarding uncertainty as to what fraction of the population has equal or lower exposures. Conversely, for any given percentile of the population, there is uncertainty as to the estimated exposure. Both one-dimensional and two-dimensional methods are demonstrated in the case-study of Annex 2.

5.2.3.1 Statistical methods based upon empirical data

Statistical methods that are based upon analysis of empirical data without prior assumptions about the type and parameter of distributions are typically termed "frequentist" methods, although sometimes the term "classical" is used (e.g. Morgan & Henrion, 1990; Warren-Hicks & Butcher, 1996; Cullen & Frey, 1999). However, the term "classical" is sometimes connoted with thought experiments (e.g. what happens with a roll of a die) as opposed to inference from empirical data (DeGroot, 1986). Therefore, we use the term "frequentist".

Frequentist methods are fundamentally predicated upon statistical inference based on the Central Limit Theorem. For example, suppose that one wishes to estimate the mean emission factor for a specific pollutant emitted from a specific source category under specific conditions. Because of the cost of collecting measurements, it is not practical to measure each and every such emission source, which would result in a census of the actual population distribution of emissions. With limited resources, one instead would prefer to randomly select a representative sample of such sources. Suppose 10 sources were selected. The mean emission rate is calculated based upon these 10 sources, and a probability distribution model could be fit to the random sample of data. If this process is repeated many times, with a different set of 10 random samples each time, the results will vary. The variation in results for estimates of a given statistic, such as the mean, based upon random sampling is quantified using a sampling distribution. From sampling distributions, confidence intervals are obtained. Thus, the commonly used 95% confidence interval for the mean is a frequentist inference based upon how the estimates of the mean vary because of random sampling for a finite sample of data.

Statistical inference can be used to develop compact representations of data sets (Box & Tiao, 1973). For example, a probability distribution model (e.g. normal, lognormal or other) can be fit to a random sample of empirical data. Examples of fitting probability distribution models to data are given in section A2.2.3 of Annex 2. The use of probability distribution models is a convenient way to summarize information. The parameters of the distributions are subject to random sampling error, and statistical methods can be applied to evaluate goodness of fit of the model to the data (Hahn & Shapiro, 1967). Goodness-of-fit methods are typically based upon comparison of a test statistic with a critical value, taking into account the sample size and desired level of significance (Cullen & Frey, 1999).

Frequentist statistical methods are powerful tools for working with empirical data. Although there appears to be a common misperception that one must have a lot of data in order to use frequentist statistics, in fact the fundamental starting point for a frequentist analysis is to have a random representative sample. Whether the data are a random representative sample depends on how the data were sampled, not on the sample size of the data. Representativeness (as defined in the Glossary) implies lack of unacceptably large bias. If one needs a random sample, and if the sample is not random, then it is also not representative. As long as this assumption is valid, it is possible to make statistical inferences even for very small data sets. The trade-off with regard to sample size is that the sampling distributions for estimates of statistics, such as the mean, distribution parameters and others, become narrower as the sample size increases. Thus, inferences based upon data with small sample sizes will typically have wider confidence intervals than those based upon larger sample sizes.

The ability to make a judgement regarding representativeness of data is closely related to data quality issues. For example, representativeness is closely associated with the data quality issue of *appropriateness*. The data quality issues of *accuracy* and *integrity* are closely related to quantification or characterization of variability and uncertainty. The data quality issue of *transparency* pertains to clear documentation that, in turn, can provide enough information for an analyst to judge the representativeness and characterize variability and uncertainty.

There are often data sets used to estimate distributions of model inputs for which a portion of data are missing because attempts at measurement were below the detection limit of the measurement instrument. These data sets are said to be censored. Commonly used methods for dealing with such data sets are statistically biased. An example includes replacing non-detected values with one half of the detection limit. Such methods cause biased estimates of the mean and do not provide insight regarding the population distribution from which the measured data are a sample. Statistical methods can be used to make inferences regarding both the observed and unobserved (censored) portions of an empirical data set. For example, maximum likelihood estimation can be used to fit parametric distributions to censored data sets, including the portion of the distribution that is below one or more detection limits. Asymptotically unbiased estimates of statistics, such as the mean, can be estimated based upon the fitted distribution. Bootstrap simulation can be used to estimate uncertainty in the statistics of the fitted distribution (e.g. Zhao & Frey, 2004). Imputation methods, such as those based on the Gibbs sampler, can be used to impute missing values for more general types of missing data.

In situations where the available data are not a random sample, the analyst is forced to make a judgement as to whether to proceed with a frequentist analysis. It may be possible to stratify the data into groups, each of which may more reasonably be assumed to be a random sample. For example, if a data set is composed of a mixture of processes (e.g. different designs within an emission source category), then it would be appropriate, if possible, to separate the data with respect to the different designs and to analyse each design separately (Zheng & Frey, 2004). However, in some cases, the data are inherently biased with respect to an assessment objective. For example, suppose that one wants to quantify the ambient concentrations of pollutants to which adults are exposed when they are outdoors. Typically, available monitoring data are collected only at a sparse set of monitoring stations and at altitudes that are not representative of the breathing zone. Thus, the uncritical use of such data could lead to biased inference as to the concentrations of pollutants to which people are actually exposed at locations and altitudes different from those of the monitoring stations. In this situation, an air quality model could be calibrated to the monitoring data and used to interpolate (or extrapolate) to other locations and altitudes. However, there would be uncertainty associated with the model prediction, in addition to measurement uncertainty associated with the available monitoring stations.

Analysts often refer to data as being "limited". In common, practical usage, the term "limited" might refer to any of several deficiencies, such as small sample size, lack of precision, lack of accuracy or lack of knowledge of the pedigree of the data. These limitations are related to the data quality concepts of accuracy and integrity. Depending on the type of limitation, the data quality problems can translate into implications for uncertainty or can lead to a representativeness problem.

Some common situations that analysts face are the following:

- **Data are a random, representative sample** of the scenario and situation of interest. In this case, the analyst can use frequentist statistical methods.

- **Data are not random but are representative in other ways**. This may mean, for example, that the data are a stratified sample applicable to the real-world situation for the assessment scenario of interest. In this case, frequentist methods can be used to make inferences for the strata that are represented by the data (e.g. particular exposed subpopulations), but not necessarily for all aspects of the scenario. However, for the components of the scenario for which the data cannot be applied, there is a lack of representative data. For example, if the available data represent one subpopulation, but not another, frequentist methods can be applied to make inferences about the former, but could lead to biased estimation of the latter. Bias correction methods, such as comparison with benchmarks, use of surrogate (analogous) data or more formal application of expert judgement, may be required for the latter.

- **Data are representative, but have other limitations**. The other limitations may include (for example) significant measurement errors, leading to lack of accuracy and precision of each measurement. In the case of lack of accuracy of measurements, bias corrections gleaned from measurements of known quantities may be useful. In the case of lack of precision, there should be recognition that the variance of the sample of measurements may be significantly larger than the variance of the true variability in the quantity, because the observed variance includes contributions from both the true variability and the additional random error inherent in the measurement technique. Thus, methods for separating measurement error from inherent variability may be required (e.g. Zheng & Frey, 2005).

- **Data are numerous but not representative**. Data do not become more representative simply by being more numerous. If the data are not for the quantity of direct interest to the assessment, the use of such data can lead to biased estimates regardless of the quantity of such data. Thus, a judgement is required (and should be explained) as to whether to use such data. If such data are used, consideration (and explanation) should be given as to why they are selected for use, the possible biases associated with inferences from such data in the context of the analysis and how such biases can be, or are, corrected in the assessment. For example, it may be known that the mean value is low because some benchmark data are available for comparison, or there are known omissions in the activity pattern or other characteristics that generated the data. In such cases, one might use the available data to gain insight into the relative range of variation compared with the observed mean value, but adjust the entire distribution to a different mean value using combinations of surrogate data, detailed analysis and expert judgement.

In situations in which the data are not a representative sample, careful consideration needs to be given to the possibility of biases. A sample would be non-representative, for example, if it were obtained for conditions or situations different from those that are assumed in the analysis. For example, suppose that emissions were measured during steady-state full-load operation, but that one desired to make predictions of emissions during transient part-load operation. The available sample of data is not representative of the desired scenario. If inferences are made based upon such data without any correction or adjustment, it is possible that the mean emission rate will be biased and that the range of variation in emissions will be incorrectly estimated.

As Morgan & Henrion (1990) point out, for many quantities of interest in models used for decision-making, there may not be a relevant population of trials of similar events upon which to perform frequentist statistical inference. For example, some events may be unique or in the future, for which it is not possible to obtain empirical sample data. Thus, frequentist statistics are powerful with regard to their domain of applicability, but the domain of applicability is limited compared with the needs of analysts attempting to perform studies relevant to the needs of decision-makers.

5.2.3.2 Methods for propagating variance or distributions through models

There are many methods and software available to assist the analyst in propagating information regarding probability distributions for inputs to a model in order to quantify key statistics of the corresponding distributions of model outputs. Here, we focus on methods that are quantitative and probabilistic. There are other quantitative methods that are not probabilistic, such as interval methods and fuzzy methods, as mentioned in sections 5.2.1 and 5.2.2, respectively. In addition, the case-study of Annex 2 mentions the factorial design method, which produces stratified quantitative estimates but does not produce a probability associated with each estimate. Annex 2 also mentions the DPD method, which is a highly granular approximation of how to stratify the probability distribution of a model output into a small number of discrete ranges.

The key methods that are the focus of this section are categorized as analytical versus numerical methods. Analytical methods can be solved using explicit equations. In some cases, the methods can be conveniently applied using pencil and paper, although for most practical problems, such methods are more commonly coded into a spreadsheet or other software. Analytical methods can provide exact solutions for some specific situations. Unfortunately, such situations are not often encountered in practice. Numerical methods require the use of a computer simulation package. They offer the advantage of broader applicability and flexibility to deal with a wide range of input distribution types and model functional forms and can produce a wide variety of output data.

Analytical and numerical methods are described in more detail below.

1) Analytical methods

Analytical methods include exact solutions for specific situations and approximate solutions that are applicable to a broader set of input distributions and model functional forms.

Exact analytical solutions can be obtained for summations of normal distributions. The sum of normal distributions is identically a normal distribution. The mean of the sum is the sum of the means of each input distribution. The variance of the sum is the sum of the variance of the inputs. Any statistic of interest for the output can be estimated by knowing its distribution type and its parameters. For example, for a model output that is a normal distribution with known parameter values, one can estimate the 95th percentile of that output.

Similarly, exact solutions can be obtained for products (or quotients) of lognormal distributions (e.g. Burmaster & Thompson, 1995). This situation may be possible for some simple exposure assessments if one is working with one equation, such as the product of intake rate, concentration in the intake media (e.g. air, liquid), exposure duration and exposure frequency, divided by an averaging time and body weight, as long as all of the input distributions are lognormal.

The exact solutions are not valid if any of the model inputs differ from the distribution type that is the basis for the method. For example, the summation of lognormal distributions is not identically normal, and the product of normal distributions is not identically lognormal. However, the Central Limit Theorem implies that the summation of many independent distributions, each of which contributes only a small amount to the variance of the sum, will asymptotically approach normality. Similarly, the product of many independent distributions, each of which has a small variance relative to that of the product, asymptotically approaches lognormality.

A method known as "transformation of variables" can be used to obtain exact analytical solutions in some situations other than those described here (Hahn & Shapiro, 1967), but is not used in practice. In practice, exposure models typically include both sums and products, such as for a multipathway exposure model. Furthermore, the inputs are not all of the same type of distribution. Also, there may be other complications, such as various types of dependencies among input distributions.

For more complex models or for input distributions for which exact analytical methods are not applicable, approximate methods might be appropriate. Many approximation methods are based on Taylor series expansion solutions, in which the series is truncated depending on the desired amount of solution accuracy and whether one wishes to consider covariance among the input distributions (Hahn & Shapiro, 1967). These methods often go by names such as "generation of system moments", "statistical error propagation", "delta method" and "first-order methods", as discussed by Cullen & Frey (1999).

The goal of approximation methods is to estimate the statistical moments of a model output based on the statistical moments of a model input. Such moments typically include the mean and variance, but can also include higher-order moments related to skewness and kurtosis (flatness of the probability distribution function). Thus, these methods do not actually quantify specific percentiles of the model output distribution. Instead, the analyst can use the estimated moments for the model output to select an appropriate parametric distribution that approximates the unknown distribution of the model output, and then any statistic of interest can be estimated for the model output. The choice of an appropriate distributional approximation of a model output can be informed by the use of a "moment plane", which is a display of regions of skewness and kurtosis that are characterized by specific types of distributions. For example, the normal distribution appears as a single point on such a plane, because it has only one possible shape. A lognormal distribution appears as a line on a plot of kurtosis versus the square of skewness, because it can take on many different magnitudes of skewness, and its probability distribution function becomes increasingly "pointy" as the skewness increases (thereby increasing the kurtosis). More details on the use of moment planes are given in Hahn & Shapiro (1967) and Cullen & Frey (1999).

Approximation methods can be useful, but as the degree of complexity of the input distributions or the model increases, in terms of more complex distribution shapes (as reflected by skewness and kurtosis) and non-linear model forms, one typically needs to carry more terms in the Taylor series expansion in order to produce an accurate estimate of percentiles of the distribution of the model output. Thus, such methods are often most widely used simply to quantify the mean and variance of the model output, although even for these statistics, substantial errors can accrue in some situations. Thus, the use of such methods requires careful consideration, as described elsewhere (e.g. Cullen & Frey, 1999).

2) Numerical methods

Numerical methods for propagating distributions through models are typically preferred over analytical methods in practice because they are versatile. Such methods can be used with a wide variety of model functional forms, including large "black box" computerized models, and for a wide variety of probability distributions used to present model inputs. However, such methods require iterative evaluation of a model, which can be computationally demanding. In some cases, it may not be feasible to do many iterations with a particular model because of large run times for just one iteration, not to mention hundreds or thousands of iterations. Of course, as computing power increases with time, models that formerly seemed dauntingly time consuming to run may be executable in minutes or seconds. Thus, the feasibility of the application of numerical methods tends to improve over time, although it also appears to be the case that as computing power increases, there is a tendency to build bigger models.

The most commonly discussed numerical method for propagating distributions through a model is Monte Carlo simulation. Monte Carlo simulation has been around for over 50 years. In practice, Monte Carlo simulation is based on generating a set of "pseudo-random" numbers for each probabilistic model input. Pseudo-random numbers should conform to an ideal of being statistically independent from one realization to another and being a sample from a uniform distribution. They should not be autocorrelated, and there should be no cycles or periodicity in the simulated numbers. A good random number generator should be able to produce millions or more such numbers before the cycle repeats. The sequence of numbers only appears to be random; in fact, the same sequence can be reproduced by setting the same "seed" values for the pseudo-random number generator each time. Thus, it is possible to reproduce the same Monte Carlo simulation at different points in time or to use the same series of random numbers to do comparisons between two options or risk management alternatives.

Monte Carlo simulation can involve several methods for using a pseudo-random number generator to simulate random values from the probability distribution of each model input. The conceptually simplest method is the inverse cumulative distribution function (CDF) method, in which each pseudo-random number represents a percentile of the CDF of the model input. The corresponding numerical value of the model input, or fractile, is then sampled and entered into the model for one iteration of the model. For a given model iteration, one random number is sampled in a similar way for all probabilistic inputs to the model. For example, if there are 10 inputs with probability distributions, there will be one random sample drawn from each of the 10 and entered into the model, to produce one estimate of the model output of interest. This process is repeated perhaps hundreds or thousands of times to arrive at many estimates of the model output. These estimates are used to describe an empirical CDF of the model output. From the empirical CDF, any statistic of interest can be inferred, such as a particular fractile, the mean, the variance and so on. However, in practice, the inverse CDF method is just one of several methods used by Monte Carlo simulation software in order to generate samples from model inputs. Others include the composition and the function of random variable methods (e.g. Ang & Tang, 1984). However, the details of the random number generation process are typically contained within the chosen Monte Carlo simulation software and thus are not usually chosen by the user.

Monte Carlo simulation is based on random sampling. Thus, it is possible to use frequentist statistical methods to estimate confidence intervals for the simulated mean of a model output, taking into account the sample variance and the sample size. Therefore, one can use frequentist methods to establish criteria for how many samples to simulate. For example, one may wish to estimate the mean of the model output with a specified precision. The number of iterations of the Monte Carlo simulation can continue until the simulation achieves convergence with the desired precision. Alternatively, a user can make an initial run of an arbitrary sample size and then do statistical analysis of the output to determine if enough runs have been made. If not, more runs can be made and combined with the data from the first set of runs, until a large enough total sample size is obtained to achieve the desired numerical precision for the model output. These types of methods are described in more detail elsewhere (e.g. Morgan & Henrion, 1990).

However, a potential pitfall of Monte Carlo simulation is becoming fixated on achieving a high degree of numerical simulation precision while losing sight of the quality of the input data. For example, if an assessment is based on model input assumptions for which there are key data quality limitations, it may not make sense to make hundreds of thousands or millions of iterations in order to obtain a highly precise numerical estimate of the model output. In some cases, analysts spend perhaps too much time and effort worrying about achieving a high degree of precision for the 99.9th percentile of a model output, when the shape and parameters of the model input distributions are not known with a high degree of confidence.

A commonly used alternative to Monte Carlo simulation is Latin hypercube sampling. Latin hypercube sampling is a stratified sampling method. In Latin hypercube sampling, a choice must be made prior to starting the simulation regarding the desired sample size. For each input, the probability distribution is divided into the specified number of equal probability ranges, according to the desired sample size. One sample is drawn from each of these equal probability ranges. Thus, each range is sampled once without replacement. Within each equal probability range, the sample can be based on the median value or can be chosen at random. The former is referred to as median Latin hypercube sampling, and the latter as random Latin hypercube sampling. One such sample is drawn for each model input that has a distribution, and one iteration of the model output is estimated. This process is repeated until all of the equal probability ranges of the inputs have been sampled. The advantage of Latin hypercube sampling over Monte Carlo simulation is that one can obtain a more stable and precise estimate of the empirical CDF of the model output in a smaller number of model iterations than for Monte Carlo simulation. However, because Latin hypercube sampling is not a random sampling method, frequentist sample statistical methods cannot be applied to characterize the precision of the output or to assist in choosing a sample size. However, ordinal statistical methods can be of some assistance in these regards (e.g. Morgan & Henrion, 1990). A potential pitfall of Latin hypercube sampling is that there may be spurious correlations among the model inputs unless a restricted pairing method is used to choose the order in which samples are drawn from the equal probability strata of each input distribution. However, numerical methods for imposing independent sampling or for inducing a specified rank correlation between two or more inputs are available (e.g. Iman & Conover, 1982).

5.2.3.3 Statistical methods based upon judgement

An alternative to the frequentist approach to statistics is based upon the use of probability to quantify the state of knowledge (or ignorance) regarding a quantity. This view is known as the personalist, subjectivist or Bayesian view (Morgan & Henrion, 1990). For consistency throughout the text, we will use the term "Bayesian". Unlike a frequentist approach, a Bayesian approach does not require assumptions about repeated trials in order to make inferences regarding sampling distributions of statistical estimates (Warren-Hicks & Butcher, 1996). Bayesian methods for statistical inference are based upon sample information (e.g. empirical data, when available) and a prior distribution. A prior distribution is a quantitative statement of the degree of belief a person has that a particular outcome will occur. For example, an expert might express a judgement regarding the distribution of fish consumption for a village composed of subsistence fishers, based upon logical inferences or analogies with other data (e.g. Cullen & Frey, 1999). Because the prior distribution expresses the state of knowledge of a particular expert (or group of experts), this distribution is conditional upon the state of knowledge. Methods for eliciting subjective probability distributions are intended to produce estimates that accurately reflect the true state of knowledge and that are free of significant cognitive and motivational biases.

Morgan & Henrion (1990) provide a useful introduction to the potential pitfalls of eliciting expert judgement regarding distributions and regarding expert elicitation protocols that are designed to overcome or minimize such pitfalls.

The cornerstone of Bayesian methods is Bayes' Theorem, which was first published in 1763 (Box & Tiao, 1973). Bayes' Theorem provides a method for statistical inference in which a prior distribution, based upon subjective judgement, can be updated with empirical data, to create a "posterior" distribution that combines both judgement and data. As the sample size of the data becomes large, the posterior distribution will tend to converge to the same result that would be obtained with frequentist methods. In situations in which there are no relevant sample data, the analysis can be conducted based upon the prior distribution, without any updating.

Although Bayesian methods are attractive with regard to their capability to accommodate information based upon both data and judgement, there appear to be several reasons for the lack of more widespread use of these methods, as described by Smith et al. (1996). Bayesian analysis is complex and requires considerable judgement and choices pertaining to prior distributions and modelling approaches. Further, software is needed to deal with complex integrations. Smith et al. (1996) argue that the frequentist methods are practical and relatively simple, although certainly there can be complex frequentist methods of inference that require judgement and software to implement.

Other often-cited drawbacks of Bayesian methods are that they are inherently subjective, and therefore there is the potential for lack of consistency or replicability, particularly if the same analysis is repeated by different groups that obtain judgements from different experts. In response, proponents of Bayesian methods typically argue that, in such situations, frequentist statistical inference cannot be applied. Although differences in judgement are to be expected among experts, sensitivity analysis methods can be used to assess whether such differences have a significant impact on the results of the analysis. If they do, then it is useful to pinpoint the source of disagreement for purposes of informing the decision-maker or to develop a research programme to collect data based on which such differences can be resolved.

While the Bayesian approach explicitly acknowledges the role of judgement, the frequentist approach also involves judgement regarding the assumption of a random, representative sample, selection of probability models, evaluation of models using specific goodness-of-fit or diagnostic checks and other steps in the analysis (e.g. Cullen & Frey, 1999).

Thus, despite its limitations, the Bayesian approach is more flexible in dealing with situations in which data are limited or not available, but in which the state of knowledge is adequate to support judgements regarding prior distributions.

5.2.4 Sensitivity analysis

Sensitivity analysis quantifies the variation in model output that is caused by specific model inputs. As such, it can be used as an underlying basis for uncertainty analysis as well as for supplying supplemental information (e.g. Cullen & Frey, 1999; Saltelli et al., 2000). Sensitivity analysis can be used to answer the following types of questions (Mokhtari & Frey, 2005):

- What is the rank order of importance among the model inputs?
- Are there two or more inputs to which the output has similar sensitivity, or is it possible to clearly distinguish and discriminate among the inputs with respect to their importance?
- Which inputs are most responsible for the best (or worst) outcomes of the output?
- Is the model response appropriate?

Sensitivity analysis can and should be used both iteratively and proactively during the course of developing an exposure model or a particular analysis. For example, sensitivity analysis can be used early in model development to determine which inputs contribute the most to variation in model outputs, to enable data collection to be prioritized to characterize such inputs. Furthermore, analysis of the model response to changes in inputs is a useful way to evaluate the appropriateness of the model formulation and to aid in diagnosing possible problems with a model. Thus, sensitivity analysis can be used to guide model development.

As part of an analysis with an existing model that has already undergone development and evaluation or when applying a newly evaluated and accepted model to a case-study, sensitivity analysis can be used to identify key sources of uncertainty that should be the target of additional data collection or research and to identify key sources of controllable variability that can be the focus of risk management strategies.

Sensitivity analysis can be either qualitative or quantitative. In a qualitative analysis, the assessor identifies the uncertainties affecting the assessment and forms a judgement of their relative importance. Such an evaluation is implicit in the qualitative approaches to assessing uncertainty, described in section 5.1. This is subjective and therefore less reliable than a quantitative sensitivity analysis. However, it is a practical first step for identifying the most important uncertainties as a focus for quantitative analysis.

Quantitative methods of sensitivity analysis and metrics for measuring sensitivity are widely available. The most commonly used sensitivity analysis methods are often relatively simple techniques that evaluate the local linearized sensitivity of model response at a particular point in the input domain. This type of approach is typically used if the model inputs are treated as point estimates, often representing the "best guess" as to the true but unknown value of each input. The sensitivity analysis of point estimates is often done for the purpose of evaluating how much the model would respond to a unit change in the input. One example is the use of partial derivatives. A simple variation on this approach is to vary each individual input over a possible range of its values, rather than just for a small perturbation or a change of only one unit of measure. Although conceptually simple, local sensitivity analysis techniques typically suffer from two key shortcomings: (1) they do not take into account the simultaneous variation of multiple model inputs; and (2) they do not take into account any non-linearities in the model that create interactions among the inputs.

If uncertainty analysis is thought of as a forward propagation of distributions through the model, then sensitivity analysis could be conceptualized as looking back from the output to the inputs to determine which of the inputs is most important to the range and likelihoods of the final result. For a probabilistic analysis based upon Monte Carlo simulation, a variety of statistically based methods can be used to ascertain what portion of the variation in the model output can be attributed to each of the model inputs. Depending on the functional form of the model, the resulting measures of sensitivity may be exact or may be approximate; however, even in the latter situation, they are typically highly informative with regard to management and planning needs. For example, because uncertainty arises from lack of perfect knowledge of the true but typically unknown value of actual emissions, uncertainty can be reduced by obtaining better information. Therefore, insights regarding key sources of uncertainty can be used to assess priorities for collecting additional data or information in order to reduce uncertainty. Sensitivity analysis is typically used to (1) assist in verification/evaluation of models, (2) identify key sources of variability and uncertainty and (3) evaluate the importance of key assumptions during model development (Russel & Dennis, 2000).

According to Mokhtari & Frey (2005), sensitivity analysis methods are typically categorized based on their scope, applicability or characteristics. Frey & Patil (2002) classify sensitivity analysis methods with regard to their characteristics as mathematical, statistical and graphical methods. Saltelli et al. (2000) classify sensitivity analysis methods with respect to their application and scope as screening, local and global. The former approach is used here.

Examples of mathematical methods include nominal range sensitivity analysis (Cullen & Frey, 1999) and differential sensitivity analysis (Hwang et al., 1997; Isukapalli et al., 2000). Examples of statistical sensitivity analysis methods include sample (Pearson) and rank (Spearman) correlation analysis (Edwards, 1976), sample and rank regression analysis (Iman & Conover, 1979), analysis of variance (Neter et al., 1996), classification and regression tree (Breiman et al., 1984), response surface method (Khuri & Cornell, 1987), Fourier amplitude sensitivity test (FAST) (Saltelli et al., 2000), mutual information index (Jelinek, 1970) and Sobol's indices (Sobol, 1993). Examples of graphical sensitivity analysis methods include scatter plots (Kleijnen & Helton, 1999) and conditional sensitivity analysis (Frey et al., 2003). Further discussion of these methods is provided in Frey & Patil (2002) and Frey et al. (2003, 2004).

Sensitivity analysis methods can be used in combination with methods for variance propagation. For example, Cullen & Frey (1999) describe how variance in the sum of random numbers can be apportioned among the inputs to the sum. All of the statistical sensitivity methods mentioned above can be applied to the results of Monte Carlo simulation, in which simulated random values are available for a model output and each probabilistic model input. FAST is an alternative method for both propagating distributions through a model and estimating the contribution of each input to the variance of the output based on a specific type of sensitivity index. Sobol's method requires some additional simulations but can be implemented in the context of Monte Carlo simulation. Guidance on how to choose sensitivity analysis methods for application to risk-related problems is given by Mokhtari & Frey (2005) and Frey et al. (2004).

> **Principle 6**
>
> *Sensitivity analysis should be an integral component of the uncertainty analysis in order to identify key sources of variability, uncertainty or both and to aid in iterative refinement of the exposure model.* The results of sensitivity analysis should be used to identify key sources of uncertainty that should be the target of additional data collection or research, to identify key sources of controllable variability that can be the focus of risk management strategies and to evaluate model responses and the relative importance of various model inputs and model components to guide model development.

5.3 Data and resource requirements

Human exposure assessments require data and models to address a number of key relationships. Here we consider the requirements for data for establishing both the structure and the numerical value of these links. Human exposures to environmental emissions include at least five important relationships that will demand data, modelling and evaluation resources:

1) the magnitude of the source medium concentration—that is, the level of contaminant that is released to indoor or outdoor air, soil, water, etc. or the level of contamination measured in or estimated in the air, soil, plants and water in the vicinity of the source;
2) the contaminant concentration ratio, which defines how much a source medium concentration changes as a result of transfers, degradation, partitioning, bioconcentration and/or dilution to other environmental media before human contact;
3) the level of human contact, which describes (often on a body weight basis) the frequency (days per year, minutes per day, etc.) and magnitude (cubic metres of air breathed per hour, kilograms of food ingested per day, square metres of surface contacted per hour, etc.) of human contact with a potentially contaminated exposure medium;
4) the duration of potential contact for the population of interest relating to the fraction of lifetime during which an individual is potentially exposed; and
5) the averaging time span for the type of health effects under consideration; that is, one must consider the appropriate averaging time span for the cumulative duration of exposure such as a human lifetime (which is typical for cancer and chronic diseases) or some relatively short time span (in the case of acute effects).

These factors typically converge as a sum of products or quotients to define a distribution of population exposure or a range of individual exposures. The reliability of population exposure estimates will depend strongly on the quantity and accuracy of the obtainable data associated with these five links.

5.4 Interpretation of results

The interpretation of uncertainty analysis results can cover a wide range of issues. Here, we consider the interpretation of results with regard to the needs of decision-makers who would use the results of uncertainty analysis in exposure assessment. The discussion is primarily based upon Morgan & Henrion (1990), Bloom et al. (1993) and Thompson & Graham (1996). The discussion is organized on the basis of key questions that decision-makers often ask, as reported by Bloom et al. (1993), based upon a survey of senior risk managers at the USEPA, and as described by Thompson & Graham (1996):

- **What is the distribution of exposures among different members of an exposed population?** This question is based upon the premise that each individual in an exposed population is expected to have different exposures because of interindividual variability in exposure factors, such as intake rate and activity patterns. If there are substantial differences in exposures among members of an exposed population, then one might identify subpopulations that tend to be more highly exposed and focus the development of exposure reduction policies for these groups. For example, because of differences in inherent characteristics or in activity patterns, some groups such as children or the elderly may be more highly exposed or more susceptible to adverse effects as a result of exposures. Thus, the analysis could be stratified to focus on such groups. Interindividual variability in exposures may raise concerns about equity.

- **How precise are the exposure estimates?** This question focuses on the simultaneous, combined effect of uncertainties in all exposure factors with respect to overall uncertainty in the exposure assessment. This question can be answered by propagating uncertainty estimates for exposure model inputs through the exposure model. Typically, this question could be answered in terms of absolute or relative ranges (e.g. a 95% probability range of ±25% of the exposure for a particular percentile of interindividual variability), based upon estimates of uncertainty for a particular percentile of the exposed population.

- **How precise do exposure estimates need to be?** The required degree of precision of an estimate will vary depending upon its intended use. For example, the degree of precision expected of a refined exposure analysis that accounts for interindividual variability is typically higher than that for a conservative screening analysis based upon upper-bound assumptions. Furthermore, the desired precision (or lack of uncertainty) would depend upon whether the range of uncertainty is large enough to cause ambiguity regarding the preferred decision. In this latter case, ideally it would be desirable to reduce uncertainty by collecting more data or information. On the other hand, some decisions may need to be made before uncertainties can be further reduced. Thus, the desirable precision might be a long-term goal but not achievable in the time frame required for a near-term decision. Recognition that management of exposure problems can be iterative and adapted over time is one strategy for reducing uncertainties in the longer term.

- **What is the pedigree of the numbers used as input to an exposure assessment?** This question deals with issues of who developed the numbers, how they were developed and who has reviewed them. For example, have they been subject to scientific peer review? Are the numbers based upon measurements, or are these preliminary estimates based upon the judgement of an analyst? The decision-maker is interested in the degree of confidence assigned to a number. This relates to concerns over whether the data were obtained using approved or acceptable measurement techniques and whether they pertain to a random representative sample of emission sources. Alternatively, data may have been obtained using a variety of measurement methods that may not be directly comparable and might be for non-representative conditions. Thus, the data may be "bad" in some way or incomplete.

- **What are the key sources of uncertainty in the exposure assessment?** This question can also be posed as: Which exposure factors contribute the most to the overall uncertainty in the inventory? This insight can be used, in turn, to target resources to reduce the largest and most important uncertainties. There are various ways to answer this question, including various forms of sensitivity analysis. For example, in the context of a probabilistic uncertainty simulation for an overall exposure assessment, various statistical methods can be used to determine which input distributions are responsible for contributing the most to the variance of the output.

- **How should efforts be targeted to improve the precision of exposure estimates?** Knowledge of key sources of uncertainty in exposure estimates helps guide additional data collection to reduce uncertainty in order to improve the precision of the estimates. For example, the identification of key sources of uncertainty can be used to prioritize information-gathering efforts for the most important inputs. Because uncertainty results from lack of knowledge, an effective approach to its reduction is to obtain more knowledge, through additional measurements or the development of more precise and accurate measurement methods.

- **How significant are differences between two alternatives?** This question pertains to determining whether it is possible to discriminate between two alternative estimates even though they are both uncertain. For example, when comparing exposure reduction strategies, does one offer high confidence of a real exposure reduction compared with a baseline even though both the estimates of baseline and controlled exposures are subject to uncertainty? This question can be answered by estimating the probability distributions for *differences* in exposures.

- **How significant are apparent trends over time?** One approach for answering this question is to evaluate the statistical significance of changes over time or to determine whether a time-series model could be used to describe data and, therefore, to gain insight regarding stationarity (or lack thereof) of the series, as well as its cycles and seasonality. Stationarity refers to a situation in which the mean and other statistics do not change as a function of time. Cycles and seasonality refer to periodicity in the time series, such as diurnal or annual effects. Comparisons of distributions for specific points in time (e.g. comparison of weekday versus weekend ambient concentrations) can also provide insight into temporal trends. For example, a probability distribution of the change in emissions from one time period to another can be used to assess the probability that emissions have increased or decreased and the likelihood of various magnitudes of the change.

- **How effective are proposed control or management strategies?** This question could pertain to the confidence with which a standard will be met. For example, Hanna et al. (2001) assess the uncertainty associated with estimates of predicted ambient ozone levels subject to a particular emission scenario, and Abdel-Aziz & Frey (2004) evaluate the probability of non-compliance with United States National Ambient Air Quality Standards for ozone based upon uncertainty in emission inventories that are propagated through an air quality model. A probability distribution of estimated exposures can be compared with a point estimate of an exposure benchmark in order to determine the probability that the benchmark will be exceeded and, if so, by how much.

- **Is there a systematic error (bias) in the estimates?** Systematic error, or bias, typically occurs when inferences are made on the basis of data that are not representative of the real-world situation for which an estimate is desired. For example, to estimate the inhalation exposures for ambient air pollution caused by power plant emissions, one has to define a scenario. The scenario might focus on actual operations of power plants for a specific time period (e.g. one year) for a particular geographic area (e.g. a state or a province). In order to estimate exposure for this scenario, one should have data representative of the particular mix of power plant designs, fuels, operating practices, loads and ambient conditions. However, if data are available only for full-load operation of plants that differ somewhat in design, fuel, operation and ambient conditions, then the average emission factor derived from the available data may differ from the true population average for the scenario of interest. The question regarding whether systematic error exists is difficult to answer in the absence of an independent basis for comparison of the estimate with some type of a "ground-truth" or "reality check". However, it is possible to incorporate expert judgements regarding sources of bias.

- **Is there ongoing research that might fill critical data gaps within the near term?** This question (and many of the others) is fundamentally motivated by the desire not to be unpleasantly surprised or overtaken by events. For example, if new research might resolve some of the key uncertainties in the assessment, is it worth waiting until that information is available before making a decision?

- **Are the estimates based upon measurements, modelling or expert judgement?** This question pertains to the pedigree of information used to support the assessment. While there is typically a preference for estimates based upon directly relevant measurements, the use of models and judgements may be justified when relevant data are not available. For example, available data may not be representative, and thus inferences based upon them may lead to biases. Moreover, there may be gaps in available data such that it is not possible to make empirically based estimates for some inventory inputs that might be critical to the assessment. In such cases, inferences could be made based upon indirect evidence (e.g. by interpolation, extrapolation or the use of theoretical hypotheses using models, or elicitation of judgement regarding subjective probability distributions for the inputs to an analysis, or both).

The preceding identification and discussion of key questions posed by decision-makers highlight the importance of identifying and characterizing uncertainty. The broad range of questions illustrates the importance of knowing what questions must be answered before developing inventories and estimates of their uncertainties. Some sources of uncertainty, such as possible sources of bias and problems with lack of data, may have to be dealt with qualitatively (e.g. by listing caveats or by using qualitative ratings) or by using expert judgement as the basis for quantifying subjective probability distributions. Other sources of uncertainty may be amenable to quantification using statistical methods based upon analysis of empirical data. Furthermore, uncertainty analysis can be supplemented with sensitivity analysis in order to identify key sources of uncertainty for purposes of prioritizing activities that could reduce uncertainty.

5.5 Use of uncertainty analysis in evaluation and validation

The USEPA's Committee on Regulatory Environmental Models defines model (or data) evaluation as

> the process for generating information over the life cycle of the project that helps to determine whether a model and its analytical results are of a quality sufficient to serve as the basis for a decision. Model quality is an attribute that is meaningful only within the context of a specific model application. In simple terms, model evaluation provides information to help assess the following factors: (a) How have the principles of sound science been addressed during model development? (b) How is the choice of model supported by the quantity and quality of available data? (c) How closely does the model approximate the real system of interest? (d) How well does the model perform the specified task while meeting the objectives set by [quality assurance] project planning? [Pascual et al., 2003]

In the context of evaluation, an uncertainty analysis

> investigates the effects of lack of knowledge and other potential sources of error in the model (e.g., the "uncertainty" associated with model parameter values) and when conducted in combination with sensitivity analysis allows a model user to be more informed about the confidence that can be placed in model results. [Pascual et al., 2003]

Validation is the process by which the reliability and relevance of a particular approach, method or assessment are established for a defined purpose (IPCS, 2004). Uncertainty analysis can contribute to this, by indicating the reliability of the exposure estimate (how different the true exposure might be) and hence its usefulness for decision-making.

An especially useful form of validation is where the results of an assessment can be compared with independent data or information (e.g. comparing predicted exposure with biomarker measurements or epidemiological studies). When making such comparisons, it is important to remember that both sides of the comparison are subject to uncertainty. The methods described in this document should be applied to the independent data, as well as to the exposure assessment, to provide a fair comparison between the two.

Adequate documentation of all aspects of the uncertainty analysis for the exposure assessment is also critical to ensure transparency to reviewers and stakeholders. This includes sufficient documentation to enable independent replication of results and necessitates detailed description of qualitative and quantitative aspects pertaining to data, scenarios, methods, inputs, models, outputs, sensitivity analysis and interpretation of results.

Transparency of documentation is also critical to adequate review of the uncertainty analysis by peers, an integral component of a defensible process for exposure and risk assessment. Selected peer reviewers must have representative expertise, which may include, but may not necessarily be limited to, analysts, exposure assessors, statisticians, etc.

It is also important to recognize that, wherever possible, characterization of exposure and associated uncertainties as a basis to define critical data gaps necessarily involves an iterative process, whereby the assessment is refined upon acquisition of additional data or evolution of methodology.

> **Principle 7**
>
> *Uncertainty analyses for exposure assessment should be documented fully and systematically in a transparent manner, including both qualitative and quantitative aspects pertaining to data, methods, scenarios, inputs, models, outputs, sensitivity analysis and interpretation of results.*

> **Principle 8**
>
> *The uncertainty analysis should be subject to an evaluation process that may include peer review, model comparison, quality assurance or comparison with relevant data or independent observations.*

> **Principle 9**
>
> *Where appropriate to an assessment objective, exposure assessments should be iteratively refined over time to incorporate new data, information and methods to better characterize uncertainty and variability.*

5.6 Summary of uncertainty characterization methods

Methods available for analysing uncertainties fall into three broad types: qualitative, deterministic and probabilistic. They provide contrasting ways of characterizing the relative importance of the uncertainties affecting an assessment and of characterizing the overall uncertainty of the assessment output, and they provide an essential input for decision-making.

In general, probabilistic approaches require more expertise and time than deterministic and qualitative approaches. For this reason, it is efficient to adopt a tiered approach, which starts by considering all uncertainties qualitatively (Tier 1). This may be sufficient, if the outcome is clear enough for risk managers to reach a decision. Otherwise, the uncertainties that appear critical to the outcome may be analysed deterministically (Tier 2) or probabilistically (Tier 3).

A range of alternative methods exists at each tier, each with its own advantages and disadvantages. Although there is substantial experience with uncertainty analysis in some fields (e.g. climate change), it would be premature to make prescriptive recommendations on which methods to use in exposure assessment. For example, when discussing the use of probabilistic methods for microbial risk assessment, the former European Commission Scientific Steering Committee concluded that "a quick harmonisation at the present state-of-the-art should be avoided" (EC, 2003). The same is true of qualitative approaches. Instead, it is desirable to maintain a flexible approach, selecting the most suitable methods for each assessment (e.g. Mokhtari & Frey, 2005). More guidance and harmonization may be possible in the longer term, as further experience accumulates.

6. COMMUNICATION

Communication about exposure and risk is difficult, partly because the information that needs to be communicated is sometimes complex, and partly because perception and evaluation of risk are influenced by a range of other factors, including the context and preconceptions of the audience. The aim of risk communication should be to supply people with the information they need to make informed decisions about risks to their health, safety and environment (NRC, 1996). Furthermore, it is generally necessary for those performing exposure assessment to communicate with several different audiences that each require different communication formats—for example, scientists, decision-makers, media and the lay public. People process information within the context of their existing "mental models" (Morgan et al., 1992) and beliefs. Dealing with exposure assessment models and corresponding results at the same time as communicating the inherent uncertainties makes the task complex. Terms such as variability between individuals and uncertainty about appropriate scenarios, models and data as well as aspects of confidence in communication partners play a central role.

6.1 Introduction and historical background

The process of risk assessment was first formalized (NRC, 1983) by the United States National Academy of Sciences through its National Research Council in 1983. The three stages of risk analysis are defined as risk assessment, risk management and risk communication (Figure 10). The important principle is the functional and organizational separation of exposure and risk assessment from risk management to avoid any non-science-driven influences on the assessment procedures. However, many interactive elements are essential for a systematic risk assessment and management process.

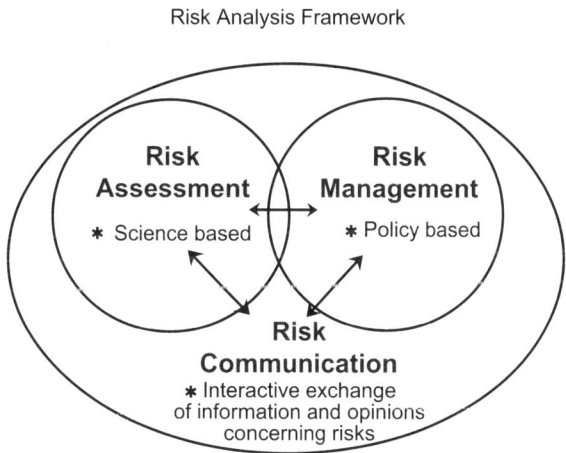

Figure 10: The relationship between the three components of risk analysis (from WHO, 2005)

What is needed for risk communication is a conceptual framework (Covello & Merkhofer, 1993) that includes at least (1) a convenient language for communication between risk assessors and risk managers, (2) a means for clarifying similarities and differences in the capabilities, applicabilities, input requirements and analytical perspectives of different assessment methods and possible consequences of restrictions, (3) a means for identifying adequate and effective methods for analysing exposure problems and (4) an aid in identifying weak links in the sequence of the exposure assessment process.

NRC (1989) defines risk communication as an interactive process of information exchange between individuals, groups and institutions. It mostly includes statements, news and messages about the nature of risks, fears and anxiety, opinions, reactions with respect to risk statements and institutional forms of risk management. Risk communication does not end at the departure gate of organizations. It is driven by a large set of attributes that influence the risk perception and the reaction to risks (Brehmer, 1987; Renn, 2005): personal control, voluntary versus involuntary, habituation to the risk, expectancy of the non-interruptable character of sequences of events, ability of perceptual recognition of the risk, irreversibility of the consequences, unfair distribution of risks and benefits, natural origin versus risks attributable to human activities, identification of the person or organization (blame) causing the risk and trust in risk regulation organizations or institutions.

Mainly in response to the anthrax attacks in the United States, in 2002, the Centers for Disease Control and Prevention published a report entitled *Crisis and Emergency Risk Communication* (Reynolds, 2002). The report illustrates two prerequisites for successful risk communication: *credibility* and *trust*. These two elements (Figure 11) may be highly important when dealing with uncertainty in exposure and risk assessment (Sjöberg, 2001). The prerequisites for credibility are accuracy of information and speed of release; the main attributes of trust are empathy and openness.

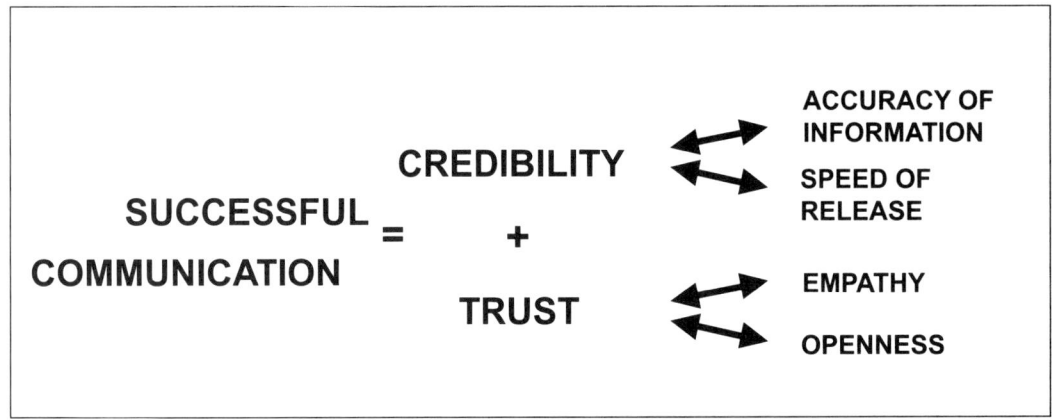

Figure 11: Elements of a successful communication (modified from Reynolds, 2002)

Accuracy of information is a result of scientific expertise, the delivery of adequate, complete and unbiased information about results and residual uncertainties. The *speed of release* is influenced by the organizational culture, to what extent the process to find answers and to acknowledge uncertainties is developed. *Empathy* is related to the willingness to recognize the situation (the scenario) in which the persons/clients are found. The degree of *openness* corresponds to the information given about uncertainties and limitations in the exposure assessment, the restrictions with respect to selected scenarios, the model assumptions and parameters for the target population, mainly the degree of possible over- and under-estimation. These aspects correspond directly to the main characteristics of uncertainty discussed in section 5.1.2.2: the appraisal of the knowledge base and the subjectivity of choices. As in any applied science, trust in the credibility of scientists dealing with complex systems (Jungermann et al., 1995) is a major influence factor for acceptance of the results.

6.2 The position of exposure and uncertainty assessment in the risk communication process

The product of the exposure assessment process should provide the scientific basis for risk management and communication, which are often initiated by identifying possible hazards. As a measurement, the result is complete only when accompanied by a quantitative statement of its uncertainty (Taylor & Kuyatt, 1994), which is required in order to decide whether the result is adequate for its intended purpose and to ascertain whether it is consistent with other similar results. In 2002, the European Commission's Health and Consumer Protection Directorate-General published a scheme in a report on animal health that highlights the role played by exposure assessment in risk assessment and emphasizes the need for risk communication in all steps of risk assessment (EC, 2002).

Risk characterization has a central position in the linkage of facts about the hazards, the choice of adequate exposure scenarios, data and assumptions, resulting in exposure calculations. The results and their inherent uncertainties give the input to the risk and consequence assessment. The risk and uncertainty assessment is intended to give "complete information to risk managers, specifically policy-makers and regulators, so that the best possible decisions are made" (Paustenbach, 1989: p. 28). Thus, the inherent uncertainties in exposure assessment will have a high impact on the management of risks. Morgan & Henrion (1990) divided those involved in the assessment and communication process roughly into groups that are (1) substance-focused, i.e. that try to obtain answers to formulated questions and to develop insight and understanding, (2) position-focused, i.e. that provide arguments and substantiation and generate answers for justification, (3) process-focused, i.e. that persuade others that things are under control and that organizations are fulfilling laws and expectations, and (4) analysis-focused, i.e. that seek professional enjoyment and reward and the development of analytical techniques.

6.2.1 Uncertainty in exposure assessment as a prognostic technique

Exposure assessment is done under the strong assumptions that (1) an adequate model for exposure calculation is on hand and (2) sufficient data about all influential exposure factors are available. The calculation is a prognosis about the expected level of exposure or the burden. Direct methods of exposure assessment, such as personal sampling (air, radiation), duplicate studies (nutrition) and human biomonitoring, provide information on a measurement level. The exposure assessors and the risk managers should balance the reasons for using prognostic techniques instead of direct exposure measurement methods. Both should anticipate critical questions about the validity of the exposure assessment technique in the course of public risk communication. Questions heard by the authors from concerned persons include, for example:

- "How sure are you about ....?"
- "What about the statement of the scientist ...., who argues ....?"
- "Did you ever prove before that your method works well?"
- "What does your method/what do your results mean for me/my family?"
- "What would be the result if you use your sophisticated model for me?"
- "Why do you use national reference data for us, aren't we different ....?"
- "Your data seem to be fairly old fashioned, doesn't the situation/product change?"

All questions deal with relevant aspects of uncertainty. The important criterion common to all these questions is the degree of structural and predictive validity (Shylakhter, 1994) of the exposure assessment.

An argument often heard in administrative units in favour of exposure assessment in contrast to biomonitoring and epidemiology is "time and costs", although it has a low impact in convincing the public, the media and other scientists. If the methods of exposure assessment have not been extensively evaluated previously, if they are new as a field application or if they have not been reviewed in an organized scientific process, doubts about the certainty, validity and objectivity should be admitted. A high level of scientific agreement is necessary for an exposure assessment approach to reach a concrete situation that is modelled by a given exposure scenario (WHO, 1999). Model-based exposure assessment is only one, normally the fastest and often the only possible step to achieve some degree of knowledge, but it uses a prognostic technique with inherent uncertainty.

6.2.2 From scenario definition to uncertainty analysis: communication with the risk managers

For the risk communication process, it is necessary that the selected scenarios for which an exposure assessment is conducted address the assessment objectives. Restrictions and limitations should be discussed and documented. Choosing a very broad scenario might lead to a lack of precision for subgroups; selecting specific groups (e.g. stratification for children, consumer habits) will result in specified models that might not be compatible with an approach for the general population. Each supplementary analysis of the possible effects of changing the scenario, the age groups, population characteristics and the model structure might show specific uncertainties, but together they secure the overall result.

The calculated exposure results are expressed in the language of numbers. The level of uncertainty is described qualitatively or quantitatively. A numerical approach has the advantages of precision, leaving less room for misinterpretation and providing more input for the decision-maker (Covello & Merkhofer, 1993).

Although numerical descriptions are usually preferred, there is a great difference between using numbers for individual predictions for persons or as an average or quantile-related estimate for the description of groups. In risk communication, both figures must be distinguished clearly; the first points to individuals, the second to aggregates (groups, communities, populations). Communication with individuals requires an individual prediction of exposure and perhaps an exposure characterization (distribution or range) of the total population for comparison. Uncertainties that might be topics of discussion are exposure events and history, day-to-day variation and questions of the inclusion of all exposure routes and pathways. For communication with groups, the presentation of the exposure assessment should mainly reflect the variability over persons and subgroups.

> Take away variety and nothing remains but averages with zero standard deviations and central tendencies always on the mark. Take away variety, in other words, and we eliminate uncertainty ... But the sum and substance of risk management is in the recognition of variety. [Bernstein, 1996]

Managers, especially those from regulatory and administrative units, seem to prefer verbal conclusions and statements in a qualitative form. This is not based on a general dislike for numbers; rather, their task is driven by such questions as "Is there enough safety for the total population or for special groups?", "Should we expect to see an exposure higher than an acceptable/legitimate level?" or "Does the exposure and risk analysis give rise to exposure reduction actions, warnings, consumer advice or prevention programmes?" All these questions contain qualities instead of quantities, and they include an evaluation of the results (and the reported uncertainty). A tiered approach with a two-dimensional Monte Carlo uncertainty analysis is useful for separating the uncertainty into uncertainty due to population variability, uncertainty due to measurement errors as well as uncertainty due to lack of knowledge. Knowing where the main contributions to uncertainty stem from allows risk managers to efficiently allocate calculated resources for the reduction of uncertainty.

As a consequence of different demands, risk managers and interested groups sometimes tend to answer by simplifications that are not acceptable to those doing exposure, uncertainty and risk assessment. Simple messages might and should be given if the scenario-related exposure assessment indicates, on Tier 1, that the probability of unwanted or unacceptably high exposure levels is very low. If it is to be expected that exposure levels for specific groups (e.g. with specific consumption or behavioural habits) may be high, then this information should be added. These answers inevitably imply a value judgement about the significance or acceptability of the exposure. To provide this goes beyond the scope of exposure assessment in two important ways: First, one cannot judge the significance of exposure without considering the dose–response relationship; and second, one cannot decide on acceptability or the need for management action without balancing the predicted effects against other factors, such as cost, benefits, new risks induced by action/reaction, social values, feasibility of control/enhancement actions, etc. The Codex Working Principles for Risk Analysis (Codex, 2005) say explicitly that it is the job of the risk manager to resolve the impact of uncertainty on decision-making, and that uncertainty should be quantified as far as scientifically achievable. In the present context, this implies that the output of the exposure assessment should—as far as possible—be quantitative. We also need to say how to communicate those uncertainties that we are unable to quantify, and this has to be done in such a way that the decision-maker can weight these unquantified uncertainties (see section 6.3.3) together with the quantified ones (see section 6.3.2).

Using default values, the selected range of the influencing variables must be chosen well, as the complaint of any particular person that "You have not considered that for me/my family the exposure (this influence factor) is higher than the one that you have used!" might devalue the whole exposure assessment in a public debate. Furthermore, in the authors' experience, it is much better to use distributions for the influence factors. Considering combinations of distributions for the input variables might lead to answers like "We have considered (foreseen) your situation, and your personal situation is included in the expected variability" or "The calculation is done as a possible combination of all (including the possible but unwanted) conditions."

Sensitivity and extreme value analysis as well as an analysis of variance propagation might lead to deeper insight into the exposure process. These steps of exposure analysis might have a particularly high value for risk management, as they identify the most influential factors and routes for high-exposure circumstances. A sensitivity analysis might clarify which influence the variance within each variable has on the variance of the target variable. If variables prove to show a low sensitivity, the influence of existing uncertainty in these variables on the result (e.g. low sample size, no knowledge of the distribution type and parameters) will be low. Risk managers will look first and foremost at variables that might be influenced (exposure frequency, concentrations). The results of a well conducted sensitivity analysis might lead directly to recommendations for exposure reduction or prevention measures, which might be justified by the state of knowledge (model) and facts (input data). Sensitivity analysis is particularly useful for an identification of the main exposure sources as well as for the selection of possible actions. It reduces uncertainty in decision-making. The knowledge gained in this step of uncertainty analysis might have a high profit in risk communication.

All this is easily written but difficult and time-consuming work to do. If "time until a first answer should/must be given" is a constraint or the "speed of release" is a critical dimension (Reynolds, 2002), then simplification is inescapable. The degree of uncertainty in exposure estimates consequently increases. It is the responsibility of exposure assessors to inform risk managers about the possible consequences of any simplification and reduction of complexity in the uncertainty of the results and the restrictions towards the generalizability of results. From the point of view of a risk manager, this might result in a crucial conflict with the exposure assessors. The result of an adequate exposure assessment includes a numerical estimate, a sensitivity analysis, an evaluation and an explanation of uncertainties. This takes time. The responsible risk manager has to decide early on the necessity of actions. Horton's (1998) paper on the precautionary principle points to this conflict:

> We must act on facts, and on the most accurate interpretation of them, using the best scientific information ... That does not mean that we must sit back until we have 100% evidence about everything. Where the state of the health of the people is at stake, the risks can be so high and the costs of corrective action so great, that prevention is better than cure. We must analyse the possible benefits and costs of action and inaction.

Consequently, risk managers, as transmitters of information to the public, want to avoid vagueness and press for precise statements (without uncertainty), as otherwise they must decide and act under uncertainty. One task of the exposure assessment step is to articulate the main arguments for restrictions with respect to the interpretation together and propose what could and should be done to enhance the scientific basis for a refined analysis that would result in less uncertainty.

6.2.3 Anticipating the demands of the audiences

NRC (1989) defined the group of players as individuals, groups and institutions. The WHO report on food safety (WHO, 1995) focuses mainly on organizational interaction "among risk assessors, risk managers, and other interested parties". Risk communication is done on all levels of interaction. In each situation, there might be a different assembly of organizations, coalitions and individuals engaged in risk communication (Figure 12), each with different communication cultures, different interests and different abilities to be articulate and participate (Gray et al., 1994). Since the process of information exchange requires a common system of symbols, signs and language, communication will depend on age, sometimes sex, education, current subject knowledge, cultural norms, language, experience and prejudice and bias—on all sides of the communication process.

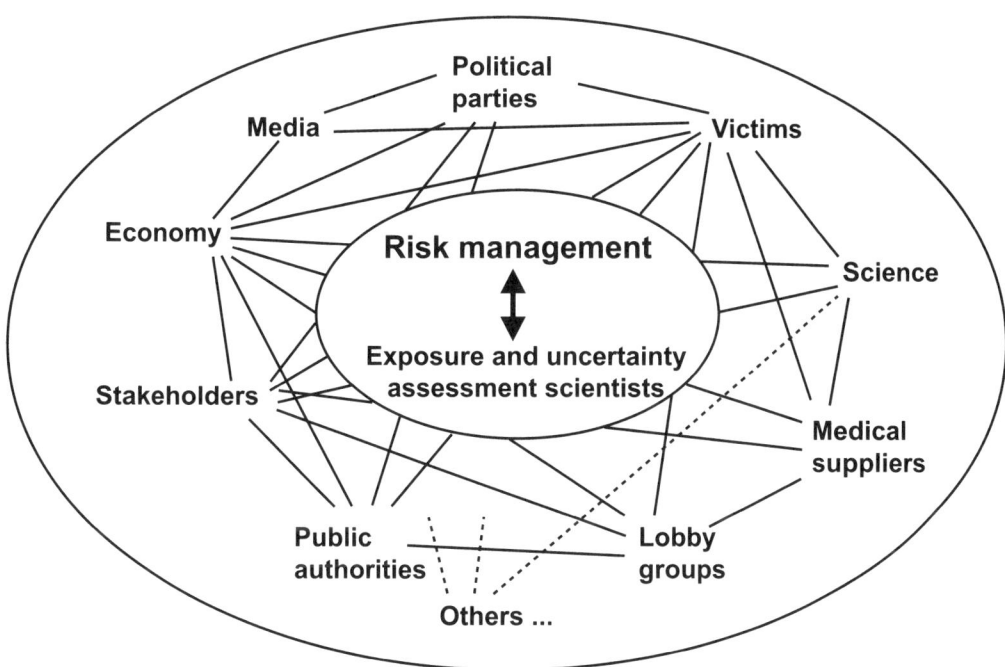

Figure 12: Communication about exposure and risk: A selection of possible actors and alliances surrounding those doing exposure assessment and uncertainty analysis

The exclusion of the lay public from informed decision-making with respect to uncertainty by the exclusive usage of an incomprehensible language violates at least the "right to know". As a consequence, information exchange and risk communication often work only with the use of informed translators (mediators). The media as well as the other participants have their own rules and habits that are rarely similar to those of the individuals doing exposure and uncertainty assessment. Risk communication should support the social and political processes of managing risks in democratic societies. Consumers react to existing uncertainties; lay people make personal decisions over which they exercise individual control (habits, preference and behaviour) and participate in democratic government processes (Morgan et al., 1992) by which decisions are made about risk issues over which individuals can exercise relatively little control (technology and industrial development, food production, exposure and risk limits). In the context of exposure assessment for specific sites, lay people are often better experts for the regional environment (related to exposure), the specific exposure conditions (scenarios) and the exposure history than are educated exposure scientists.

6.2.4 Requirements for accepted exposure assessment

Clearness and transparency with respect to the choice of models, methods, assumptions, distributions and parameters are two prerequisites for trust and confidence; openness about uncertainties is another. Exposure assessment as an applied science should follow the main scientific desiderata: empirical testing, documentation and reproducibility of results, explicit reporting of uncertainty, peer review and an open debate about underlying theories and models. This way, the main attributes for characterizing uncertainty discussed in the last chapter, the appraisal of the knowledge base and the subjectivity of choices, are clarified.

Even if adequate documentation exists, a complete and thorough peer review of exposure models can be an extremely time-consuming and difficult business. Model assessment should include a reanalysis of all input data, assumptions and models, as well as an examination of all simplifications, formulas, computer codes and programming features, together with additional runs of the models to examine sensitivities and hidden bugs (GAO, 1979). Exposure models as complex models are implemented in special programming languages or spreadsheets. Problems in reviewing exposure models might arise from the code testing alone (Panko, 1998; Henrion, 2004).

> It is unrealistic to expect a reviewer to be able to perform a complete assessment, unpaid and single handed. In the case of large models, a proper external assessment will require a multidisciplinary team, and a significant budget. [Morgan & Henrion, 1990: p. 20]

Point and range estimates as well as probabilistic models (Monte Carlo simulation) must show complete reproducibility per programming environment, since the underlying algorithms are deterministic. They should show asymptotic equivalence of results over different software environments and simulation techniques.

6.3 Proposals for the presentation/visualization of uncertainty

The presentation of results should support an unbiased understanding of the results of the exposure assessment to enable the members of the target groups to make informed and independent decisions. This requires a basic understanding of the exposure process (the model from source to dose/burden) and at least an intuitive competence to understand the quantitative data and results in nature and magnitude. The selected scenario, data, model assumptions, results and inherent uncertainties should be communicated in an understandable and scientifically accepted presentation format. Presentations should be tailored to address the questions and information needs of the different audiences. To handle the different levels of sophistication and detail needed, it may be useful to design a presentation in a tiered format where the level of detail increases with each successive tier (USEPA, 1997b).

6.3.1 Presentation of numerical results

Textual descriptions of the exposure assessment results might be useful if statements about the mean, the central tendency estimate (median) or a selected quantile of the exposure distribution are given without a description of uncertainty. However, each of the point estimates mentioned will have a different level of uncertainty with respect to model assumptions, database and calculation method. A typical wording to describe results might be, for example:

> Taking into account the restrictions/the uncertainty/the lack of sufficient data/…, we assume/expect/calculate/ …that the exposure of the population/of the most exposed group/the highest exposed individual/...
> - is in the range from … to … (for x%)
> - is lower than … for 95%/99%/… of the population
> - is lower than … with … % confidence

A textual presentation of results should in no way lead to a mixture of verbal descriptions of numerical results with an evaluation of results. In 2000, the European Commission gave this clear advice:

> … the Scientific Committees should be aware that adjectives such as minimal, negligible, etc. and expressions as "no risk", "acceptable risk", etc. may sound to have a different meaning for scientists, experts and the layman. The glossary could explain the exact meaning attributed to these expressions or, alternatively, each opinion should explain the exact context in which such expressions are used. In general, judgements about "acceptability" ought to be used only when clear legislative terms of reference are available … otherwise the criterium [sic] of acceptability should be explained in detail. In every case, it seems to be very important that the reader is informed about existence or non-existence of official EU legislation of reference within the frame of which the risk assessment judgement is formulated. [EC, 2000: p. 174]

Although the advice is given mainly for the description of risk assessment results, it holds completely for exposure assessment, since the quantitative input for risk assessment is exposure assessment and uncertainty analysis. Since any description of the resulting exposure distribution(s) in terms such as "very low", "low", "fair", "moderate", "high" or "extreme" includes an evaluation, it must be defined and justified (EnHealth Council, 2004). Those communicating the results of an exposure assessment frequently use comparative reporting schemes, such as "the {*50%/majority/ … /95%*} of {*data/measurements/individuals*} show exposure {*values/estimates/measurements*} lower than the {*tolerable daily intake (TDI)/reference dose (RfD)/acceptable daily intake (ADI)/ … /target value/reference value/limit value*} or "The exposure {*value/estimate/measurement*} is about x% of the {*TDI/RfD/ADI/ … /target value/reference value/limit value*}". Statements of this type are incomplete without a reference to the regulatory authority, without a definition of the target group (adults, children) and without an explicit documentation of the applied value. If possible, an uncertainty range of the exposure incidence rate (in per cent) that is expected to show values higher than the chosen cut-off value should be added as a numerical documentation or as a verbal description. Comparative evaluation of results without reporting the results of the assessment will not support the credibilty of the reported results. In general, it will be difficult to give a simple textual description of the expected variability in exposure results together with a description of the influence of uncertainty in a mainly textual format (Budescu & Wallsten, 1995).

The presentation of results in graphical formats is "state of the art" (USEPA, 2000). Although we do not have uniformly accepted recommendations for the presentation formats, the targets of the visualization approaches seem to be in accordance with the following criteria to describe the expected variability in the target population:

- description of the full range of the exposure distribution by displaying a cumulative density and a density function of the distribution;
- control for the cumulative probability distribution (per cent under/over a given value);
- description of the central tendency (mean and median = 50th percentile); and
- description of selected percentage values (1st, 5th and/or 95th, 99th percentiles) for which the population exposure is under/over the given percentiles.

Alternative approaches using box and whisker plots, pie charts and different types of visualizations of density functions are discussed in Ibrekk & Morgan (1987) and Morgan & Henrion (1990). Each has advantages for specific tasks, but the performance of a display depends upon the information that a subject is trying to extract (central tendency or variation).

The visualization of uncertainty within the graphical presentation formats introduces an additional dimension in the display. In the simplest form, this is displayed by a set of corresponding confidence intervals or grey/colour shadings around the central tendency estimate function(s). This is discussed in the following section. Substantial interaction with end users (mostly risk assessors) suggests that it is helpful to get the audience accustomed to one type of graph first before exposing them to the many possible variations; cumulative distributions seem to be a good first choice (especially when one wants to show confidence intervals around the distribution; this does not work well with probability distribution functions). If the audience will accept two types of graph, cumulative distributions are good for quantities where the interest is in small values (e.g. toxicity), and inverse cumulative distributions (exceedance plots) are better where the interest is in high values (e.g. exposure, frequency of impacts). A display of the density function adds information about the shape and the modal values of the distribution (see Figure 13 in the next section).

6.3.2 Communication of quantified uncertainties[2]

Communicating uncertainty adds complexity, because it involves communicating ranges or distributions of possible risks, rather than single estimates. However, research studies indicate that the majority of people do understand the difference between interval and point estimates of risk (Johnson & Slovic, 1995, 1998). Among those respondents who understood the concept, reporting of uncertainty had mixed effects (Johnson, 2003). On one hand, discussion of uncertainty appeared to signal more honesty. On the other hand, discussion of uncertainty led to lower competence ratings of the institutions responsible for risk assessment. Graphical

---

[2] The text in section 6.3.2 has been published in similar form in EFSA (2006), because the two documents were developed in parallel involving communication between the two processes and the experts involved.

presentation of uncertainty produced higher comprehensibility ratings, but lower trustworthiness ratings. The potential for such responses needs to be considered by scientists and risk managers when deciding how to communicate with consumers. However, the main focus in this section is on finding effective ways for scientists to communicate uncertainty to risk managers.

Routine assessments account for uncertainty by using standard factors and assumptions. In these cases, it is sufficient to give the result, state that the standard factors were applied and refer the reader to other sources (e.g. an official guidance document) for the derivation and justification of those factors. If there could be questions about the applicability of the standard factors to the case in hand (e.g. for a novel contaminant), then the decision to use them should be justified.

Uncertainties assessed at Tier 1 (qualitative) may be communicated by listing or tabulating them, together with an indication of their direction and magnitude. Possible formats for this are illustrated in chapter 5. In addition, it will generally be desirable to give a more detailed textual discussion of the more important uncertainties in the list and of their combined effect on the assessment outcome.

Uncertainties assessed at Tier 2 (deterministic) generate alternative point estimates for exposure and may be communicated in various ways, depending on the particular methods used for sensitivity analysis. As a minimum, this should identify which sources of uncertainty have been treated at Tier 2, state and justify the alternative quantitative estimates used for each one (e.g. minimum, maximum and most likely values), present exposure estimates for those combinations of alternative estimates that are considered plausible and state and justify any combinations of estimates that are considered implausible. In addition, it will be useful (especially if upper estimates exceed levels of concern) to show which of the quantified uncertainties have most influence on the outcome.

Uncertainties assessed at Tier 3 (probabilistic) produce probability distributions as outputs. Probability distributions can be communicated in many ways, including:

- probability density function, showing the relative probability of different values;
- cumulative distribution, showing the probability of values below any given level;
- exceedance (inverse cumulative) distribution, showing the probability of values above any given level; and
- summary statistics, e.g. mean or median estimates for the 97.5th percentile exposure together with one or more confidence intervals (e.g. 75%, 90%, 95% or 99% intervals). These may be presented numerically or graphically (e.g. box and whisker plots).

Examples of the three types of graphical representation are shown in Figure 13. These hypothetical examples show uncertainty distributions for the exposure of the 97.5th percentile consumer; this could equally be done for other percentiles or for the average consumer.

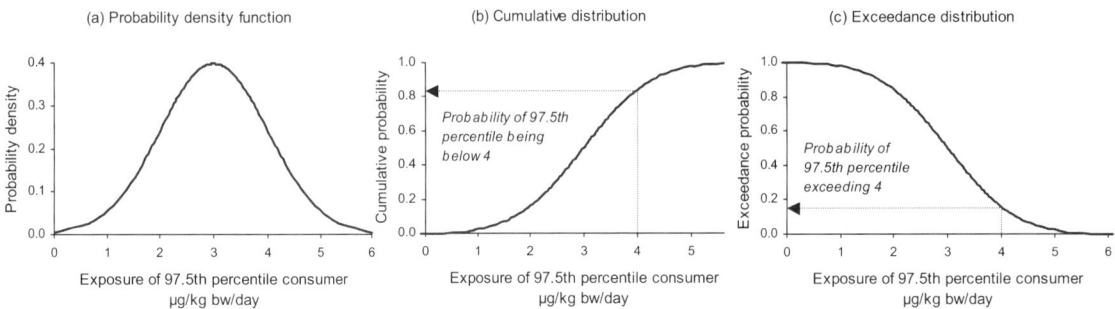

Figure 13: Examples of three different formats for presenting probability distributions. bw = body weight.

A more complex graphical format can be used to show a distribution for variability of exposure across the whole population, together with confidence intervals to show uncertainty (e.g. Figure 14). This can be used to read off confidence intervals for the exposure of any given percentile consumer.

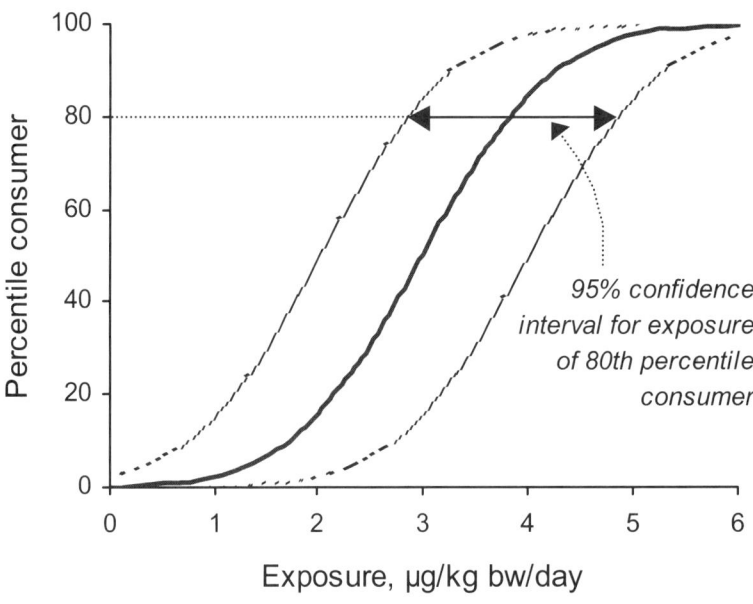

Figure 14: Example of cumulative distribution for variability of exposure between consumers (thick curve), with 95% confidence intervals (thin curves) showing uncertainty for each percentile consumer. Other confidence intervals (e.g. 90% or 99%) could be shown, depending on the level of confidence wanted by risk managers. bw = body weight.

Cumulative distributions have been found to be more intuitive for non-technical audiences than are other kinds of display (Morgan & Henrion, 1990) and are convenient for reading off different percentiles (e.g. median, 95th percentile). Cumulative distributions are especially useful when interest is focused on low values (e.g. intake of nutrients), while exceedance distributions may be more intuitive when the interest is in high values (e.g. exposure to contaminants). However, the most likely value (mode) and shape of the distribution are shown more clearly by a probability density function, and the USEPA (1997b) recommends showing both cumulative distributions and probability density functions side by side. Whatever methods are used for presenting the results, it is helpful to provide a textual explanation as well.

It is essential to provide decision-makers with an assessment of the overall degree of uncertainty in the assessment outcome. Therefore, if the uncertainties for an assessment have been analysed at different tiers (qualitatively, deterministically and probabilistically), it is necessary to find a way of presenting the results together and arriving at an overall characterization of exposure. This is difficult and subjective but unavoidable, since it is never possible to quantify all uncertainties objectively. Few assessments have attempted to do this in a systematic way, and it would be premature to give firm recommendations. However, a combined presentation should include:

- a list of the uncertainties that have been treated probabilistically (Tier 3), and appropriate graphical, numerical and textual presentation of the results;
- a list of the uncertainties treated deterministically (Tier 2), showing the results obtained with alternative assumptions; and
- a list of the uncertainties treated qualitatively (Tier 1), together with an evaluation of the direction and magnitude of their impact on the assessment outcome.

In addition, it will generally be desirable to produce a concise textual and numerical summary of the results—for example, for use in the executive summary of an exposure assessment. The appropriate format for this will vary from case to case, but one possible format for a Tier 3 assessment might be:

> The median estimate of the 97.5th percentile exposure is x, but this is affected by a number of uncertainties. Uncertainties A, B, C ... were analysed probabilistically, resulting in a $p\%$ confidence interval of y–z. This included reasonable worst-case assumptions for uncertainties D, E, F ..., which were not treated probabilistically. Evaluation of further, unquantified uncertainties suggests that the true 97.5th percentile exposure could be higher/is unlikely to be higher, because ...

Note that the choice of confidence intervals ($p\%$) to use in such statements should be agreed with decision-makers, since it implies a risk management judgement about how much certainty is required. Although 95% intervals are frequently used in biological research, a higher or lower degree of certainty may be appropriate for risk management, and the degree may vary from case to case depending on the other risks and benefits at stake.

In addition to communicating results, it is essential to communicate sufficient information about the methods used so that peer reviewers can fully evaluate them, and so that other specialists can repeat the assessment if desired. This is especially important for sensitivity analysis and probabilistic approaches, although it may be sufficient to describe them in outline if the reader can be referred to other sources for detail.

6.3.3 Communication of unquantified uncertainties

A key part is how to communicate the *unquantified uncertainties*. It is often suggested that it is good practice to list or describe the uncertainties affecting an exposure or risk assessment. Cooke (1991: p. 3) uses the fourfold distinction for the degree of science-based reasoning used in the risk communication process: "conjecture – belief – correct reasoning – knowledge". Many scientific and public heated debates about exposure and risk assessment deal with the status of arguments of the communication partners in this line. However, simply listing and categorizing uncertainty are not very helpful to the decision-maker. Chapter 3 gives an overview on how to assess the sources of uncertainty. What the decision-maker needs to know is the combined effect of the uncertainties on the assessment outcome: in other words, how different the true exposure might be. Therefore, it is desirable, even in a qualitative assessment, to give some indication of the direction and magnitude of each individual source of uncertainty and the combined effect of all the uncertainties considered.

One promising attempt to do this might be to present a table listing the unquantified uncertainties and indicating the direction and magnitude of each to indicate relative magnitude and direction of influence on risk estimate. In a second step, an overall assessment of the combined influence of the tabulated uncertainties on the risk estimate might be presented. Of course, all this represents a subjective and qualitative statement, but it has the character of a transparent visualization of an evaluation, based on the knowledge and experience of the exposure and risk expert (group). We think it will work best when the magnitudes can be expressed in relation to some decision threshold; for example, an uncertainty that might take the risk above the acceptable limit (set by risk managers) could be indicated as highly relevant. Although the approach seems to be quite simple, it might give a framework for a qualitative evaluation of the content, steps and results as a basis for a transparent discussion.

Two aspects of magnitude are worth considering. One is the relative magnitude of different sources of uncertainty, which can help to prioritize which uncertainties to reduce by collecting additional data. The other is the magnitude of the uncertainties compared with the margin between the estimated exposure and any level of concern to the risk manager (if known). This is important when considering whether the uncertainties are large enough to change the overall outcome and risk management judgement.

Clearly, any qualitative assessment of the direction and magnitude of uncertainties and of their combined influence on the assessment outcome is bound to be subjective. This makes it very dependent on the knowledge, experience and expertise of the assessor. Some might argue that this makes it inappropriate or even dangerous to do. However, the alternatives are even less attractive: leave the assessment of uncertainty to risk managers (who generally have less relevant knowledge, experience and expertise) or ignore uncertainty altogether (in which case public decisions are based on best estimates without attention to the likelihood or consequences of other outcomes). Quantification may help, but is not possible for all uncertainties. Therefore, the least bad option is to start with a qualitative assessment, interpret it cautiously to take account of its subjectivity and use it to decide whether a more quantitative assessment is needed (see section 5.1.2.2). A simple approach for this could comprise the following elements: (1) consider all parts of the model and list all identifiable sources of uncertainty, (2) subjectively evaluate any directional influence of each source of uncertainty, (3) evaluate the magnitude of each source of uncertainty on the assessment outcome, ideally relative to the relevant risk management threshold, (4) evaluate the combined influence of the listed uncertainties on the assessment outcome (direction and magnitude) and, finally, (5) if the combined influence of the uncertainties is clearly not sufficient to alter the risk management judgement, then further assessment may not be required. If, on the other hand, the combined influence indicates a sufficient probability that the risk management judgement could be altered, then a more refined assessment may be justified.

The subjectivity of the qualitative assessment (see section 5.1.2.2) also opens the possibility of conscious or unconscious bias by the assessor. For this reason, it is desirable to report the steps from (1) to (5) in a transparent way so that others can review and evaluate the judgements that have been made. This has the advantage that it is always possible to do and that it is sufficient if the result is clearly conservative (protective) overall. However, it has disadvantages with regard to subjectivity when the outcome is not clearly conservative and when using separate uncertainty factors for many parameters that can lead to compounding conservatism. If an exposure/risk assessment contains a number of conservative assumptions, then the above table is likely to end up with an overall assessment that the true risk is probably lower than the quantitative estimate. However, if the assessment attempts to use realistic estimates/distributions for most inputs, then a table of unquantified uncertainties is the likely result. This undoubtedly is a difficulty for decision-makers unless the assessor can evaluate the combined uncertainty relative to the decision-makers' decision threshold.

As a conclusion of this section about the role of uncertainty analysis and description, it is worth noting that despite all the work and effort, a scientifically adequate analysis and description of uncertainty will lead to some discomfort and might introduce an element of communication conflict. This is a consequence of the state of uncertainty and should be considered. Some people are tempted not to show the quantified and especially the unquantified uncertainties, but that does not solve the underlying problem. Since transparency is an important attribute of openness and trust, both will help to increase the confidence of those involved in dealing with risks.

6.4 Avoiding typical conflicts in risk communication

A high degree of communication between those involved in the process is a necessary but sometimes not sufficient prerequisite to avoid risk communication conflicts. Those persons who represent organizations in the communication process and especially in the public should obtain at lcast some basic understanding of the benefits and problems of exposure, uncertainty and risk assessment. However, this cannot be expected for all communication partners. If different organizations and groups with a different background of interests, faculty and profession are involved, it might be useful to plan the risk communication process. At least some types of conflicts mentioned below can be anticipated, avoided or reduced:

- *Information sharing*: Whether organizations or facilities disclose or withhold any relevant information or specific data needed for the specification and calculation of an exposure scenario, distrust and public conflict will be guaranteed. Uncertainty is seldom, if ever, an acceptable excuse for waiting to communicate or deliver risk information (Covello et al., 1988). The "right to know" all relevant information, the exposure results, the uncertainties and the risk evaluations is an important issue for organizations as well as for the public.

- *Participation*: Non-involvement in the risk communication process of those individuals, organizations and institutions that have an organizational, professional or individual interest in the risk topic might lead to distrust, multiple assessments and, later, a divergence of results and evaluations. The key actors should at least be informed and, depending on the public character of the process, invited to share the process. A lack of involvement might and often will result in conflicts/misunderstanding about the completeness or correctness of data, the methods and the appropriateness of the standards and norms used in risk evaluation.

- *Facts and methods*: Obtaining agreement in the scientific community about the selected exposure scenario, the assumptions, the models, the data, the methods and the remaining uncertainties should be an early target of any exposure assessment. Seeking consensus about the selected (sub)population, the quality of input and the model will enhance the acceptance of the results. Involving different scientific approaches and describing the existing level of uncertainty increase the quality of the assessment and might lead to an anticipation of the pro and con arguments coming in a later stage of the risk communication process. However, if the data and results are highly uncertain, some people are likely to complain that the given facts are too uncertain to trust.

- *Evaluation of results*: The result of an exposure assessment is a value or a distribution of expected exposure values, together with a range of uncertainty. If limiting values with some formal or accepted legitimation exist (laws, directives, parliamentary governmental or organizational decisions), the evaluation of the results is not in the hands of or the responsibility of the risk manager. If the evaluation of the results is carried out for new substances (hazards), the choice of the level of safety is a matter of scientific and public debate. In the second case, answers to questions such as "What is safe enough?" or "What are the safety targets?" must be found. It is the right of any individual or group to make a claim for "No exposure! No risk!". Acceptability for a burden of exposure, for uncertainty and for risks cannot be demanded by comparison with other individual risks or by cross-reference to legislation for other hazards. The evaluation of an exposure and uncertainty assessment as well as the risk regulation must follow the laws and the rules of a democratic society. Even if a justified regulation is notified, it is the right of each individual communication partner not to accept it.

- *Consequences and necessary actions*: Since it seems to be difficult to find public consensus in the evaluation of exposure assessment results, it should be expected to be more difficult to find an agreement about the necessity and the kind of actions as a consequence of the assessment results, including the uncertainty. Covello et al. (1988) state that "Often, actions are what people most want to know about. ... People want to know what you do to reduce emissions, not just how much is emitted and how many deaths or illnesses may result". In risk communication, the choice of no or adequate actions will be questioned by different groups for different targets, and uncertainty ("Will you wait until ... has happened?") might be an important argument in the demand for action.

The guiding risk communication tips of the United States Centers for Disease Control and Prevention (Reynolds, 2002)—"Don't give overassurance!", "Acknowledge uncertainty!" and "Explain the process to find the answer!"—might help sometimes to communicate uncertainty in an understandable and fair manner. Levinson (1991) advised that companies as well as organizations in general cannot improve the relationships to communication partners by risk communication alone: "The most productive way is to build trust", which might be done by exposure and risk reduction programmes (reduction of the use of toxic substances, of emissions and of hazardous waste). Organizations should develop a risk communication culture that supports this process.

> **Principle 10**
>
> *Communication of the results of exposure assessment uncertainties to the different stakeholders should reflect the different needs of the audiences in a transparent and understandable manner.*

6.5 Conclusions

As in everyday life, the credibility of the players in risk communication (individuals or organizations) plays a central role in risk communication. Credibility is a basic element of risk communication with respect to scientific correctness and transparency about the current limitations in knowledge and existing uncertainty. Social trust is the main factor in risk acceptance and risk management (Renn & Levine, 1991). Credibility of organizations, institutions and individuals can be destroyed very quickly and very efficiently (Alhakami & Slovic, 1994), and credibility develops very slowly (Bord & O'Connor, 1992). These statements might explain the credibility crisis suffered by many institutions and organizations. A change in dealing with uncertainty in exposure assessment as well as a change in communicating about it might enhance the communication process.

7. CONCLUSIONS

Part 1 of this IPCS Harmonization Project Document describes, characterizes and provides guidance for uncertainty analysis in routine exposure assessment work. It also discusses challenges and limitations, as it cannot answer all the questions that may be posed in uncertainty analysis; rather, it demonstrates that uncertainty analysis is a dynamic process.

An uncertainty analysis gives the assessor the opportunity to re-evaluate the scenario, model approaches and parameters of the analysis and to consider their influence in the overall analysis. The practical impact of uncertainty analysis is illustrated within the annexed case-studies, which also clarify how uncertainty analyses follow a systematic methodology, based on a tiered approach, and consider all possible sources of uncertainty. The first step in uncertainty analysis consists of a screening, followed by a qualitative analysis and two levels of quantitative analysis, using deterministic and probabilistic data. The assessor should be aware that an uncertainty analysis cannot answer all the questions, which, moreover, may lead to new questions.

Finally, the results of the uncertainty analysis should be adequately communicated, together with the results of the assessment. Addressing the uncertainties of the exposure assessment enables the risk assessor to distinguish risk characterization and risk assessment. Further, the results of the exposure assessment enable the risk manager to identify the key factors that influence exposures and risks.

Key guiding principles for uncertainty analysis are identified throughout the text and provided together in the Executive Summary. These guiding principles are considered to be the general desirable goals or properties of a good exposure assessment.

8. REFERENCES

Abdel-Aziz A, Frey HC (2004) Propagation of uncertainty in hourly utility NO_x emissions through a photochemical grid air quality model: A case study for the Charlotte, NC modeling domain. *Environmental Science and Technology*, 38(7): 2153–2160.

Adolf TR, Eberhardt W, Hartmann S, Herwig A, Heseker H, Matiaske B, Moch KJ, Rosenbauer J (1994) *Ergebnisse der nationalen Verzehrsstudie (1985-1988) über die Lebensmittel- und Nährstoffaufnahme in der Bundesrepublik Deutschland.* Niederkleen, Wissenschaftlicher Fachbuchverlag Dr. Fleck, Vol. XI, Verbundstudie Ernährungserhebung Risikofaktoren Analytik (VERA) Schriftenreihe.

Alhakami AS, Slovic P (1994) A psychological study of the inverse relationship between perceived risk and perceived benefit. *Risk Analysis*, 14(6): 1085–1096.

Ang AH-S, Tang WH (1984) *Probability concepts in engineering planning and design. Vol. 2. Decision, risk, and reliability.* New York, NY, John Wiley and Sons.

Bernstein PL (1996) *Against the gods: The remarkable story of risk.* New York, NY, John Wiley and Sons.

Bevington PR (1969) *Data reduction and error analysis for the physical sciences.* New York, NY, McGraw-Hill, pp. 56–65.

BgVV (2001) *Workshop on exposure of children to substances used as ingredients in pesticides.* Berlin, German Federal Ministry for the Environment, Nature Conservation and Nuclear Safety, Federal Institute for Health Protection of Consumers and Veterinary Medicine (Bundesinstitut für gesundheitlichen Verbraucherschutz und Veterinärmedizin) (Grant No. 201 61 218/01; http://www.bfr.bund.de/cm/225/exposure_of_children_to_plant_protection_agents.pdf).

Bloom DL, Byrne DM, Anderson JM (1993) *Communicating risk to senior EPA policy-makers: A focus group study.* Prepared by Bloom Research and the Office of Air Quality Planning and Standards, United States Environmental Protection Agency, Research Triangle Park, NC.

Bord RJ, O'Connor RE (1992) Determinants of risk perception of a hazardous waste site. *Risk Analysis*, 12(3): 411–416.

Box GEP, Tiao GC (1973) *Bayesian inference in statistical analysis.* New York, NY, Wiley-Interscience.

Brehmer B (1987) The psychology of risk. In: Singleton WT, Hovden J, eds. *Risk and decision.* New York, NY, John Wiley, pp. 25–39.

Breiman L, Friedman JH, Stone CJ, Olshen RA (1984) *Classification and regression trees.* Belmont, CA, Chapman & Hall/CRC Press.

Budescu DV, Wallsten TS (1995) Processing linguistic probabilities: General principles and empirical evidence. *The Psychology of Learning and Motivation*, 32: 275–318.

Burke JM, Zufall MJ, Özkaynak H (2001) A population exposure model for particulate matter: Case study results for $PM_{2.5}$ in Philadelphia, PA. *Journal of Exposure Analysis and Environmental Epidemiology*, 11: 470–489.

Burmaster DE, Thompson KM (1995) Backcalculating cleanup targets in probabilistic risk assessments when the acceptability of cancer risk is defined under different risk management policies. *Human and Ecological Risk Assessment*, 1(1): 101–120.

BVL (2006) *Lebensmittel-Monitoring*. Bonn, Federal Office of Consumer Protection and Food Safety (Bundesamt für Verbraucherschutz und Lebensmittelsicherheit) (http://www.bvl.bund.de/cln_007/DE/01__Lebensmittel/01__Sicherheit__Kontrollen/03__Monitoring/Monitoring__node.html__nnn=true).

Codex (2005) Working principles for risk analysis for application in the framework of the Codex Alimentarius. In: *Codex Alimentarius Commission procedural manual*, 15th ed. Rome, Codex Alimentarius Commission, pp. 101–107 (ftp://ftp.fao.org/codex/Publications/ProcManuals/Manual_15e.pdf).

Cohen Hubal EA, Sheldon LS, Burke JM, McCurdy TR, Berry MR, Rigas ML, Zartarian VG, Freeman NC (2000) Children's exposure assessment: A review of factors influencing children's exposure, and the data available to characterize and assess that exposure. *Environmental Health Perspectives*, 108(6): 475–486.

Cooke R (1991) *Experts in uncertainty: Opinion and subjective probability in science*. New York, NY, Oxford University Press.

Covello VT, Merkhofer MW (1993) *Risk assessment methods: Approaches for assessing health and environmental risks*. New York, NY, Plenum Press.

Covello VT, Sandman PM, Slovic P (1988) *Risk communication, risk statistics and risk comparisons: A manual for plant managers*. Washington, DC, Chemical Manufacturers Association.

Cullen AC, Frey HC (1999) *The use of probabilistic techniques in exposure assessment: A handbook for dealing with variability and uncertainty in models and inputs*. New York, NY, Plenum Press.

DeGroot MH (1986) *Probability and statistics*, 2nd ed. Reading, MA, Addison-Wesley.

EC (2000) *First report on the harmonisation of risk assessment procedures. Part 1: The report of the Scientific Steering Committee's Working Group on Harmonisation of Risk Assessment Procedures in the scientific committees advising the European Commission in the area of human and environmental health*. Brussels, European Commission, Health &

Consumer Protection Directorate-General, 26–27 October 2000 (http://ec.europa.eu/food/fs/sc/ssc/out83_en.pdf).

EC (2002) *Preliminary report on the risk assessment for animal populations.* Discussed by the Scientific Steering Committee at its meeting of 7–8 November 2002. Brussels, European Commission, Health & Consumer Protection Directorate-General (http://ec.europa.eu/food/fs/sc/ssc/out298_en.pdf).

EC (2003) Preliminary report. Risk assessment of food borne bacterial pathogens: Quantitative methodology relevant for human exposure assessment. Appendix 3 in: *The future of risk assessment in the European Union. The second report on the harmonisation of risk assessment procedures.* Brussels, European Commission, Scientific Steering Committee (http://ec.europa.eu/food/fs/sc/ssc/out252_en.pdf).

Eckhardt R (1987) Stan Ulam, John von Neumann and the Monte Carlo method. *Los Alamos Science*, 15: 131–143 (http://fas.org/sgp/othergov/doe/lanl/pubs/00326867.pdf).

Edwards AL (1976) *An introduction to linear regression and correlation.* San Francisco, CA, W.H. Freeman.

EFSA (2006) Guidance of the Scientific Committee on a request from EFSA related to uncertainties in dietary exposure assessment. *The EFSA Journal*, 438: 1–54 (http://www.efsa.europa.eu/EFSA/Scientific_Opinion/sc_op_uncertainty%20exp_en.pdf).

Emond MJ, Lanphear BP, Watts A, Eberly S, and Members of the Rochester Lead-in-Dust Study Group (1997) Measurement error and its impact on the estimated relationship between dust lead and children's blood lead. *Environmental Research*, 72(1): 82–92.

EnHealth Council (2004) *Environmental health risk assessment guidelines for assessing human health risks from environmental hazards.* Canberra, Commonwealth of Australia, Department of Health and Ageing, Population Health Division, June (http://www.health.gov.au/internet/wcms/publishing.nsf/Content/ohp-ehra-2004.htm).

EU (2002a) *Technical notes for guidance: Human exposure to biocidal products—Guidance on exposure estimation.* Ispra, European Union, European Chemicals Bureau, Directorate-General Environment, June (B4-3040/2000/291079/MAR/E2; http://ecb.jrc.it/biocides/).

EU (2002b) Human exposure to biocidal products. User guidance version 1. Annex 4 in: *Technical notes for guidance: Human exposure to biocidal products—Guidance on exposure estimation.* Ispra, European Union, European Chemicals Bureau, 76 pp. (http://ecb.jrc.it/Documents/Biocides/TECHNICAL_NOTES_FOR_GUIDANCE/TNsG_ON_HUMAN_EXPOSURE/Users_guidance_to_Report_2002.doc).

EU (2003) *Technical guidance document on risk assessment in support of Commission Directive 93/67/EEC on risk assessment for new notified substances, Commission Regulation (EC) No 1488/94 on risk assessment for existing substances and Directive 98/8/EC of the European Parliament and of the Council concerning the placing of biocidal products on the market. Part I.* Ispra, European Union, European Chemicals Bureau, Joint Research Centre, Institute for Health and Consumer Protection (EUR 20418 EN/1; http://ecb.jrc.it/tgdoc/).

EU (2005) *Work Package 1. Development of the concept of exposure scenarios. General framework of exposure scenarios. Scoping study for technical guidance document on preparing the chemical safety report under REACH, final report.* European Union, European Chemicals Bureau (REACH Implementation Project 3.2-1A Lot 1; Commission Service Contract No. 22551-2004-12 F1SC ISP BE; http://ecb.jrc.it/DOCUMENTS/REACH/RIP_FINAL_REPORTS/RIP_3.2-1_CSA-CSR_SCOPING/EXPOSURE_SCENARIOS/RIP3.2-1_WP_1_ES_Final_28072005.doc).

Evans GW, Karwowski W, Wilhelm MR (1986) An introduction to fuzzy set methodologies for industrial and systems engineering. In: Evans GW, Karwowski W, Wilhelm MR, eds. *Applications of fuzzy set methodologies in industrial engineering.* New York, NY, Elsevier, pp. 3–11.

Evans JS, Graham JD, Gray GM, Sielken RL (1994) A distributional approach to characterizing low-dose cancer risk. *Risk Analysis*, 14(1): 25–34.

Ferson S (1996) What Monte Carlo methods cannot do. *Human and Ecological Risk Assessment*, 2(4): 990–1007.

Fiserova-Bergerova V, Pierce JT, Droz PO (1990) Dermal absorption potential of industrial chemicals: Criteria for skin notation. *American Journal of Industrial Medicine*, 17: 617–635.

Frey HC, Patil R (2002) Identification and review of sensitivity analysis methods. *Risk Analysis*, 22(3): 553–577.

Frey HC, Mokhtari A, Danish T (2003) *Evaluation of selected sensitivity analysis methods based upon applications to two food safety process risk models.* Prepared by North Carolina State University for Office of Risk Assessment and Cost–Benefit Analysis, United States Department of Agriculture, Washington, DC (http://www.ce.ncsu.edu/risk/Phase2Final.pdf).

Frey HC, Mokhtari A, Zheng J (2004) *Recommended practice regarding selection, application, and interpretation of sensitivity analysis methods applied to food safety process risk models.* Prepared by North Carolina State University for Office of Risk Assessment and Cost–Benefit Analysis, United States Department of Agriculture, Washington, DC (http://www.ce.ncsu.edu/risk/Phase3Final.pdf).

GAO (1979) *Guidelines for model evaluation.* Washington, DC, United States General Accounting Office (Technical Report PAD-79-1).

Gray PCR, Biocca M, Stern RM (1994) *Communicating environment and health risks in Europe*, 5th version. Norwich, University of East Anglia, Centre for Environmental and Risk Management, pp. 354–385.

Guy RH, Potts RO (1992) Structure–permeability relationships in percutaneous penetration. *Journal of Pharmaceutical Sciences*, 81(6): 603–604.

Hahn GJ, Shapiro SS (1967) *Statistical models in engineering*. New York, NY, John Wiley and Sons.

Hanna SR, Lu Z, Frey HC, Wheeler N, Vukovich J, Arunachalam S, Fernau M, Hansen DA (2001) Uncertainties in predicted ozone concentrations due to input uncertainties for the UAM-V photochemical grid model applied to the July 1995 OTAG domain. *Atmospheric Environment*, 35(5): 891–903.

Heinemeyer G, Scholtz R, Lindtner O (2006) *Formaldehyd – Exposition und offene Fragen*. Berlin, Federal Institute for Risk Assessment (BfR) (http://www.bfr.bund.de/cm/232/formaldehyd_exposition_und_offene_fragen.pdf).

Henrion M (2004) *What's wrong with spreadsheets—and how to fix them with Analytica*. Los Gatos, CA, Lumina Decision Systems, Inc. (http://www.lumina.com/dlana/papers/Whats%20wrong%20with%20spreadsheets.pdf, accessed 10 July 2006).

Horton R (1998) The *new* new public health of risk and radical engagement. *Lancet*, 352: 251–252.

Hwang D, Byun DW, Odman MT (1997) An automatic differentiation technique for sensitivity analysis of numerical advection schemes in air quality models. *Atmospheric Environment*, 31(6): 879–888.

Ibrekk H, Morgan MG (1987) Graphical communication of uncertain quantities to nontechnical people. *Risk Analysis*, 7(4): 519–529.

Iman RL, Conover WJ (1979) The use of rank transform in regression. *Technometrics*, 21(4): 499–509.

Iman RL, Conover WJ (1982) A distribution free approach to inducing rank correlation among input variables. *Communications in Statistics*, B11(3): 311–334.

Iman RL, Shortencarier MJ (1984) *A FORTRAN 77 program and user's guide for the generation of Latin hypercube and random samples for use with computer models*. Albuquerque, NM, Sandia National Laboratories (Report Nos. SAND83-2365 and NUREG/CR-3624).

Industrial Economics, Inc. (2004) *An expert judgment assessment of the concentration–response relationship between $PM_{2.5}$ exposure and mortality*. Prepared by Industrial Economics, Inc., under subcontract to Abt Associates, Inc., for the Office of Air Quality Planning and Standards, United States Environmental Protection Agency, Research Triangle Park, NC, 23 April (http://www.epa.gov/ttn/ecas/regdata/Benefits/pmexpert.pdf, accessed 1 May 2007).

IPCC (2000) *Good practice guidance and uncertainty management in national greenhouse gas inventories.* Intergovernmental Panel on Climate Change, National Greenhouse Gas Inventories Programme (http://www.ipcc-nggip.iges.or.jp/public/gp/english/).

IPCS (2000) Human exposure and dose modelling. In: *Human exposure assessment.* Geneva, World Health Organization, International Programme on Chemical Safety (Environmental Health Criteria 214; http://www.inchem.org/documents/ehc/ehc/ehc214.htm#PartNumber:6).

IPCS (2004) *IPCS risk assessment terminology. Part 2. IPCS glossary of key exposure assessment terminology.* Geneva, World Health Organization, International Programme on Chemical Safety (IPCS Harmonization Project Document No. 1; http://www.who.int/ipcs/methods/harmonization/areas/ipcsterminologyparts1and2.pdf).

IPCS (2005a) *Chemical-specific adjustment factors for interspecies differences and human variability: Guidance document for use of data in dose/concentration–response assessment.* Geneva, World Health Organization, International Programme on Chemical Safety (IPCS Harmonization Project Document No. 2; http://whqlibdoc.who.int/publications/2005/9241546786_eng.pdf).

IPCS (2005b) *Principles of characterizing and applying human exposure models.* Geneva, World Health Organization, International Programme on Chemical Safety (IPCS Harmonization Project Document No. 3; http://whqlibdoc.who.int/publications/2005/9241563117_eng.pdf).

IPCS (2006a) *Principles for evaluating health risks in children associated with exposure to chemicals.* Geneva, World Health Organization, International Programme on Chemical Safety (Environmental Health Criteria 237; http://www.who.int/ipcs/publications/ehc/ehc237.pdf).

IPCS (2006b) *Dermal absorption.* World Health Organization, International Programme on Chemical Safety (Environmental Health Criteria 235; http://www.who.int/ipcs/publications/ehc/ehc235.pdf).

Isukapalli SS, Georgopoulos PG (2001) *Computational methods for sensitivity and uncertainty analysis for environmental and biological models.* Research Triangle Park, NC, United States Environmental Protection Agency, Office of Research and Development, National Exposure Research Laboratory, 145 pp. (EPA/600/R-01-068; http://www.ccl.rutgers.edu/reports/EPA/edmas_v3_epa.pdf).

Isukapalli S, Roy Z, Georgopoulos PG (2000) Efficient sensitivity/uncertainty analysis using the combined stochastic response surface method (SRSM) and automatic differentiation for FORTRAN code (ADIFOR): Application to environmental and biological systems. *Risk Analysis*, 20: 591–602.

Jablonowski M (1998) Fuzzy risk analysis in civil engineering. In: Ayyub BM, ed. *Uncertainty modeling and analysis in civil engineering.* Boca Raton, FL, CRC Press, pp. 137–148.

Jelinek F (1970) *Probabilistic information theory*. New York, NY, McGraw-Hill Book Company.

Johnson BB (2003) Further notes on public response to uncertainty in risks and science. *Risk Analysis*, 23(4): 781–789.

Johnson BB, Slovic P (1995) Presenting uncertainty in health risk assessment: Initial studies of its effects on risk perception and trust. *Risk Analysis*, 15(4): 485–494.

Johnson BB, Slovic P (1998) Lay views on uncertainty in environmental health risk assessments. *Journal of Risk Research*, 1(4): 261–279.

Jungermann H, Pfister H-R, Fischer K (1995) Credibility, information preferences, and information interests. *Risk Analysis*, 16(2): 251–261.

Kelvin L (1901) Nineteenth century clouds over the dynamical theory of heat and light. *The London, Edinburgh and Dublin Philosophical Magazine and Journal of Science*, 6(2): 1–40.

Khuri AJ, Cornell JA (1987) *Response surfaces*. New York, NY, Marcel Dekker Inc.

Kleijnen JPC, Helton JC (1999) Statistical analyses of scatterplots to identify important factors in large-scale simulations. 1: Review and comparison of techniques. *Reliability Engineering & System Safety*, 65(2): 147–185.

Krayer von Krauss MP, Janssen PHM (2005) Using the W&H integrated uncertainty analysis framework with non-initiated experts. *Water Science & Technology*, 52(6): 145–152.

Layton DW (1993) Metabolically consistent breathing rates for use in dose assessments. *Health Physics*, 64(1): 23–36.

Levinson A (1991) Risk communication: Talking about risk reduction instead of acceptable risk. In: Zervos C, Knox K, Abramson L, Coppock R, eds. *Risk analysis: Prospects and analysis*. New York, NY, Plenum Press, pp. 387–392.

Mekel O, coord. (2003) [*Evaluation of standards and models for probabilistic exposure assessment. Interim report.*] Bielefeld, Universität Bielefeld (Forschungs- und Entwicklungsprojekt; http://www.math.uni-bremen.de/riskom/xprob/pdfs/xprob_1_zwischenbericht.pdf) (in German).

Metropolis N, Ulam S (1949) The Monte Carlo method. *Journal of the American Statistical Association*, 44(247): 335–341.

Mokhtari A, Frey HC (2005) Recommended practice regarding selection of sensitivity analysis methods applied to microbial food safety process risk models. *Human and Ecological Risk Assessment*, 11(3): 591–605.

Morgan MG, Henrion M (1990) *Uncertainty: A guide to dealing with uncertainty in quantitative risk and policy analysis.* New York, NY, Cambridge University Press.

Morgan WG, Fischhoff B, Bostrom A, Lave L, Atman CJ (1992) Communicating risk to the public. First, learn what people know and believe. *Environmental Science & Technology*, 26(11): 2048–2056.

Mosbach-Schulz O (1999) [Methodical aspects of probabilistic modelling.] *Umweltwissenschaften und Schadstoff-Forschung – Zeitschrift für Umweltchemie und Ökotoxikologie*, 11(5): 292–298 (in German).

Neter J, Kutner MH, Wasserman W, Nachtsheim CJ (1996) *Applied linear statistical models*, 4th ed. Chicago, IL, McGraw-Hill Book Company.

NRC (1983) *Risk assessment in the federal government: Managing the process* (also known as the *Red Book*). Committee on the Institutional Means for Assessment of Risks to Public Health, Commission on Life Sciences, National Research Council. Washington, DC, National Academy Press (http://www.nap.edu/books/0309033497/html/).

NRC (1989) *Improving risk communication.* Committee on Risk Perception and Communication and Commission on Physical Sciences, Mathematics, and Applications, National Research Council. Washington, DC, National Academy Press (http://www.nap.edu/books/0309039436/html/).

NRC (1994) *Science and judgment in risk assessment.* Committee on Risk Assessment of Hazardous Air Pollutants, Board on Environmental Studies and Toxicology, Commission on Life Sciences, National Research Council. Washington, DC, National Academy Press (http://www.nap.edu/books/030904894X/html/index.html).

NRC (1996) *Understanding risk: Informing decisions in a democratic society.* Committee on Risk Characterization, Commission on Behavioral and Social Sciences and Education, National Research Council. Washington, DC, National Academy Press (http://www.nap.edu/books/030905396X/html/).

OEHHA (2000) *Air Toxics Hot Spots Program risk assessment guidelines. Part IV. Technical support document for exposure assessment and stochastic analysis.* Oakland, CA, California Environmental Protection Agency, Office of Environmental Health Hazard Assessment (http://www.oehha.ca.gov/air/hot_spots/pdf/Stoch4f.pdf).

Panko RR (1998) What we know about spreadsheet errors. *Journal of End User Computing*, 10(2): 15–21.

Pascual P, Stiber N, Sunderland E (2003) *Draft guidance on the development, evaluation, and application of regulatory environmental models.* Prepared by the Council for Regulatory Environmental Modeling, Office of Science Policy, Office of Research and Development, Washington, DC, November (http://www.epa.gov/ord/crem/library/CREM%20Guidance%20Draft%2012_03.pdf).

Paté-Cornell E (1996a) *Different levels of treatment of uncertainty in risk analysis and aggregation of expert opinions*. Presented at Elements of Change Conference, Aspen Global Change Institute, Aspen, CO, 31 July – 8 August 1996.

Paté-Cornell E (1996b) Uncertainties in risk analysis: Six levels of treatment. *Reliability Engineering & System Safety*, 54: 95–111.

Paustenbach DJ (1989) A survey of health risk assessment. In: Paustenbach DJ, ed. *The risk assessment of environmental and human health hazards: A textbook of case studies*. New York, NY, John Wiley and Sons, p. 27.

Renn O (with annexes by Graham P) (2005) *Risk governance—Towards an integrative approach*. Geneva, International Risk Governance Council (IRGC White Paper No. 1).

Renn O, Levine D (1991) Credibility and trust in risk communication. In: Kasperson RE, Stallen PJM, eds. *Communicating risks to the public—International perspectives*. Dordrecht, Kluwer, pp. 175–218.

Reynolds B, ed. (2002) *Crisis and emergency risk communication*. Atlanta, GA, Centers for Disease Control and Prevention and Agency for Toxic Substances and Disease Registry, October (http://publichealth.yale.edu/ycphp/CERCFiles/TrainerResources/CDCCERC_Book.pdf).

Ruffle B, Burmaster DE, Anderson PD, Gordon HD (1994) Lognormal distributions for fish consumption by the general US population. *Risk Analysis*, 14(44): 395–404.

Russel A, Dennis R (2000) NARSTO critical review of photochemical models and modeling. *Atmospheric Environment*, 34(12–14): 2283–2324.

Saltelli A, Chan K, Scott EM (2000) *Sensitivity analysis*. Chichester, John Wiley & Sons Ltd.

Shylakhter AI (1994) Uncertainty estimates in scientific models: Lessons from trends in physical measurements, population and energy projections. In: Ayyub BM, Gupta MM, eds. *Uncertainty modelling and analysis: Theory and applications*. Amsterdam, Elsevier Science B.V., pp. 477–496 (http://theory.csail.mit.edu/~ilya_shl/alex/94c_uncertainty_scientific_models_physical_measurements_projections.pdf).

Sjöberg L (2001) Limits of knowledge and the limited importance of trust. *Risk Analysis*, 21(1): 189–198.

Smith EP, Ye K, McMahon AR (1996) Bayesian statistics: Evolution or revolution. *Human and Ecological Risk Assessment*, 2(4): 660–665.

Sobol IM (1993) Sensitivity analysis for nonlinear mathematical models. *Mathematical Modeling and Computational Experiment*, 1(4): 407–414.

Taylor BN, Kuyatt CE (1994) *Guidelines for evaluating and expressing the uncertainty of NIST measurement results*. Washington, DC, National Institute of Standards and Technology (NIST Technical Note 1297; http://physics.nist.gov/Pubs/guidelines/cover.html, accessed 8 August 2006).

Thompson KM, Graham JD (1996) Going beyond the single number: Using probabilistic risk assessment to improve risk management. *Human and Ecological Risk Assessment*, 2(4): 1008–1034.

USEPA (1992) *Guidelines for exposure assessment*. Washington, DC, United States Environmental Protection Agency, Risk Assessment Forum (EPA/600/Z-92/001, 29 May). *Federal Register*, 57(104): 22888–22938.

USEPA (1997a) *Exposure factors handbook. Vols. I, II and III*. Washington, DC, United States Environmental Protection Agency, National Center for Environmental Assessment, Office of Research and Development, August (EPA/600/P-95/002F{a,b,c}; http://www.epa.gov/ncea/efh/).

USEPA (1997b) *Guiding principles for Monte Carlo analysis*. Washington, DC, United States Environmental Protection Agency, Office of Research and Development, March (EPA/630/RZ-97/001; http://www.epa.gov/ncea/raf/montecar.pdf, accessed 16 August 2004).

USEPA (2000) *Guidance for data quality assessment. Practical methods for data analysis*. Washington, DC, United States Environmental Protection Agency, Office of Research and Development, July (EPA/600/R-96/084; http://www.epa.gov/quality/qs-docs/g9-final.pdf).

USEPA (2001) *Risk assessment guidance for Superfund. Vol. III, Part A. Process for conducting probabilistic risk assessment (RAGS 3A)*. Washington, DC, United States Environmental Protection Agency (EPA 540-R-02-002; OSWER 9285.7-45; PB2002 963302; http://www.epa.gov/oswer/riskassessment/rags3adt/index.htm).

USEPA (2004) EPA's risk assessment process for air toxics: History and overview. In: *Air toxics risk assessment reference library. Vol. 1. Technical resource manual*. Washington, DC, United States Environmental Protection Agency, pp. 3-1 – 3-30 (EPA-453-K-04-001A; http://www.epa.gov/ttn/fera/data/risk/vol_1/chapter_03.pdf).

van der Sluijs JP, Craye M, Funtowicz S, Kloprogge P, Ravetz J, Risbey J (2005) Combining quantitative and qualitative measures of uncertainty in model-based environmental assessment: The NUSAP system. *Risk Analysis*, 25(2): 481–492.

Vuori V, Zaleski RT, Jantunen MJ (2006) ExpoFacts—An overview of European exposure factors data. *Risk Analysis*, 26(3): 831–843.

Walker WE, Harremoës P, Rotmans J, van der Sluijs JP, van Asselt MBA, Janssen P, Krayer von Krauss MP (2003) Defining uncertainty: A conceptual basis for uncertainty management in model-based decision support. *Integrated Assessment*, 4(1): 5–17.

Warren-Hicks WJ, Butcher JB (1996) Monte Carlo analysis: Classical and Bayesian applications. *Human and Ecological Risk Assessment*, 2(4): 643–649.

WHO (1995) *Application of risk analysis to food standards issues*. Report of the Joint FAO/WHO Expert Consultation, Geneva, 13–17 March 1995. Geneva, World Health Organization (WHO/FNU/FOS/95.3; http://www.fao.org/docrep/008/ae922e/ae922e00.htm).

WHO (1999) *Accepting epidemiological evidence for environmental health impact assessment*. Report of the WHO Working Group, WHO European Centre for Environment and Health (ECEH) Symposium at the International Society for Environmental Epidemiology (ISEE)/International Society of Exposure Analysis (ISEA) Conference, Athens, 4–8 September 1999.

WHO (2005) *Relationship between the three components of risk analysis*. Geneva, World Health Organization, Department of Food Safety, Zoonoses and Foodborne Diseases, 21 October (http://www.who.int/foodsafety/micro/3circles_diagram_color.jpg).

Willett W (1998) *Nutritional epidemiology*, 2nd ed. Oxford, Oxford University Press.

Wilschut A, ten Berge WF, Robinson PJ, McKone TE (1995) Estimating skin permeation: The validation of five mathematical skin permeation models. *Chemosphere*, 30(7): 1275–1296.

Xue J, Zartarian V, Özkaynak H, Dang W, Glen G, Smith L, Stallings CA (2006) Probabilistic arsenic exposure assessment for children who contact chromated copper arsenate (CCA)-treated playsets and decks. Part 2: Sensitivity and uncertainty analyses. *Risk Analysis*, 26(2): 533–541.

Zadeh LA (1965) Fuzzy sets. *Information and Control*, 8: 338–353.

Zartarian VG, Ott WR, Duan N (1997) A quantitative definition of exposure and related concepts. *Journal of Exposure Analysis and Environmental Epidemiology*, 7(4): 411–437.

Zartarian VG, Xue J, Özkaynak H, Dang W, Glen G, Smith L, Stallings C (2005) *A probabilistic exposure assessment for children who contact CCA-treated playsets and decks using the Stochastic Human Exposure and Dose Simulation model for the wood preservative exposure scenario (SHEDS-Wood). Final report*. Washington, DC, United States Environmental Protection Agency (EPA/600/X-05/009; http://www.epa.gov/heasd/sheds/CCA_all.pdf).

Zartarian V, Xue J, Özkaynak H, Dang W, Glen G, Smith L, Stallings CA (2006) Probabilistic arsenic exposure assessment for children who contact CCA-treated playsets and decks. Part 1: Model methodology, variability results, and model evaluation. *Risk Analysis*, 26(2): 515–531.

Zhao Y, Frey HC (2004) Quantification of variability and uncertainty for censored data sets and application to air toxic emission factors. *Risk Analysis*, 24(3): 1019–1034.

Zheng J, Frey HC (2004) Quantification of variability and uncertainty using mixture distributions: Evaluation of sample size, mixing weights and separation between components. *Risk Analysis*, 24(3): 553–571.

Zheng J, Frey HC (2005) Quantitative analysis of variability and uncertainty with known measurement error: Methodology and case study. *Risk Analysis*, 25(3): 663–676.

GLOSSARY OF TERMS

The terms below have been adopted or adapted from existing definitions for use in the context of human exposure assessment. Definitions of additional terms used in this document may be found in the IPCS risk assessment terminology Harmonization Project Document (IPCS, 2004).

Accuracy
Degree of agreement between average predictions of a model or the average of measurements and the true value of the quantity being predicted or measured. Accuracy is also a criterion used to evaluate the knowledge base uncertainty. It focuses on the identification of the most important bottlenecks in the available knowledge and the determination of their impact on the quality of the result.

Aleatory uncertainty
Aleatory is of or pertaining to natural or accidental causes and cannot be explained with mechanistic theory. Generally interpreted to be the same as stochastic variability.

Appraisal of the knowledge base
A characteristic of the uncertainty. It is used for qualitative characterization of the source of uncertainty. The appraisal of the knowledge base focuses on the adequacy of the available knowledge base for the exposure assessment (e.g. identification of data gaps and their impact on outcome).

Bias
Also referred to as systematic error. Difference between the mean of a model prediction or of a set of measurements and the true value of the quantity being predicted or measured.

Bootstrap simulation
A statistical technique based on multiple resampling with replacement of the sample values or resampling of estimated distributions of the sample values that is used to calculate confidence limits or perform statistical tests for complex situations or where the distribution of an estimate or test statistic cannot be assumed.

Central tendency
The central tendency of a probability distribution typically refers to the mean (arithmetic average) or median (50th percentile) value estimated from the distribution. For some very highly skewed distributions, the mean might not represent central tendency. Some analysts prefer to use the median as a central tendency estimate. For distributions that have only one mode, the modal value is sometimes considered to be a central tendency estimate.

Choice space
A criterion used to evaluate the subjectivity of choices characteristic of uncertainty. It focuses on spanning the alternative choices.

Confidence interval
An estimated two-sided interval from the lower to upper confidence limit of an estimate of a statistical parameter. This interval is expected to enclose the true value of the parameter with a specified confidence. For example, 95% confidence intervals are expected to enclose the true values of estimated parameters with a frequency of 95%.

Controllable variability
Sources of heterogeneity of values of time, space or different members of a population that can be modified in principle, at least in part, by intervention, such as a control strategy. For example, variability in emissions of a chemical to the atmosphere could be modified via a control strategy. For both population and individual risk, controllable variability is a component of overall variability.

Credibility interval
Similar to a confidence interval, except that a credibility interval represents the degree of belief regarding the true value of a statistical parameter.

Critical control point
A point, step or procedure at which control can be applied and a hazard can be prevented, eliminated or reduced to an acceptable level.

Critical limit
A criterion that must be met for each preventive measure associated with a critical control point.

Cumulative distribution function (CDF)
A quantitative representation of a probability distribution model that is obtained by integrating the probability density function. The CDF provides a quantitative relationship between the value of a quantity selected from the distribution and its corresponding cumulative probability (percentile).

Data quality objective
Expectations or goals regarding the precision and accuracy of measurements, inferences from data regarding distributions for inputs and predictions of the model.

Deterministic
An estimate that is based on a single value for each model input and a corresponding individual value for a model output, without quantification of the cumulative probability or, in some cases, plausibility of the estimate with respect to the real-world system being modelled. This term is also used to refer to a model for which the output is uniquely specified based on selected single values for each of its inputs.

Discrete probability distribution
A probability distribution for which there are discrete portions of the sample space, each of which has its own probability (or frequency). An example would be a distribution regarding the fraction of exposed persons that are members of specific age cohorts.

Distribution (normal, lognormal, uniform, log-uniform, triangular, beta, gamma, logistic, loglogistic)

A probability distribution is a mathematical description of a function that relates probabilities with specified intervals of a continuous quantity, or values of a discrete quantity, for a random variable. Probability distribution models can be non-parametric or parametric. A non-parametric probability distribution can be described by rank ordering continuous values and estimating the empirical cumulative probability associated with each. Parametric probability distribution models can be fit to data sets by estimating their parameter values based upon the data. The adequacy of the parametric probability distribution models as descriptors of the data can be evaluated using goodness-of-fit techniques. Distributions such as normal, lognormal and others are examples of parametric probability distribution models.

Epistemic

Of or pertaining to human knowledge.

Exposure route

The way in which an agent enters a target after contact (e.g. by ingestion, inhalation or dermal absorption).

Extreme value analysis

Analysis of stochastic processes for the purpose of estimating the probabilities of rare events. Such analysis is often made difficult by uncertainties in the statistics because of an inherent scarcity of data.

Goodness-of-fit test

A procedure for critiquing and evaluating the potential inadequacies of a probability distribution model with respect to its fitness to represent a particular set of observations.

Influence of choices on results

A criterion used to evaluate the subjectivity of choices characteristic of uncertainty. It determines the influence of the choices on the results.

Influence of situational limitations on choices

A criterion used to evaluate the subjectivity of choices characteristic of uncertainty. It determines the influence of situational limitations (e.g. money, tools and time) on the choices.

Inherent randomness

Random perturbations that are irreducible in principle, such as Heisenberg's Uncertainty Principle.

Inputs

Quantities that are entered into a model.

Interindividual variability

see Variability

Intersubjectivity among peers and among stakeholders
A criterion used to evaluate the subjectivity of choices characteristic of uncertainty. It focuses on both the similarity and controversy of choices among peers and among stakeholders.

Intraindividual variability
see Variability

Level of uncertainty
A characteristic of the uncertainty. It is used for qualitative characterization of the source of uncertainty. The level of uncertainty is essentially an expression of the degree of severity of the uncertainty, as seen from the assessors' perspective.

Model
A set of constraints restricting the possible joint values of several quantities. A hypothesis or system of belief regarding how a system works or responds to changes in its inputs. The purpose of a model is to represent as accurately and precisely as necessary with respect to particular decision objectives a particular system of interest.

Model boundaries
Designated areas of competence of the model, including time, space, pathogens, pathways, exposed populations and acceptable ranges of values for each input and jointly among all inputs for which the model meets data quality objectives.

Model detail
Level of simplicity or detail associated with the functional relationships assumed in the model compared with the actual but unknown relationships in the system being modelled.

Model structure
A set of assumptions and inference options upon which a model is based, including underlying theory as well as specific functional relationships.

Model uncertainty
Bias or imprecision associated with compromises made or lack of adequate knowledge in specifying the structure and calibration (parameter estimation) of a model.

Parameter
A quantity used to calibrate or specify a model, such as "parameters" of a probability model (e.g. mean and standard deviation for a normal distribution). Parameter values are often selected by fitting a model to a calibration data set.

Plausibility
A criterion used to evaluate the knowledge base uncertainty. It focuses on the completeness of the knowledge base and the acknowledgement of ignorance when applicable.

Precision
A measure of the reproducibility of the predictions of a model or repeated measurements, usually in terms of the standard deviation or other measures of variation among such predictions or measurements.

Probabilistic analysis
Analysis in which distributions are assigned to represent variability or uncertainty in quantities. The form of the output of a probabilistic analysis is likewise a distribution.

Probability
Defined depending on philosophical perspective: 1. the frequency with which we obtain samples within a specified range or for a specified category (e.g. the probability that an average individual with a particular mean dose will develop an illness); 2. degree of belief regarding the likelihood of a particular range or category.

Probability density function
A function that relates "probability density" to point values of a continuous random variability or that relates "probability" to specific categories of a discrete random variable. The integral (or sum) must equal one for continuous (discrete) random variables.

Random error
Processes that are random or statistically independent of each other, such as imperfections in measurement techniques that lead to unexplainable but characterizable variations in repeated measurements of a fixed true value. Some random errors could be reduced by developing improved techniques.

Refined method
A method intended to provide accurate exposure and risk using appropriately rigorous and scientifically credible methods. The purpose of such methods, models or techniques is to produce an accurate and precise estimate of exposure and/or risk consistent with data quality objectives and/or best practice.

Reliability
A criterion used to evaluate the knowledge base uncertainty. It focuses on the identification of the scientific status of the knowledge base and the determination of its quality soundness.

Representativeness
The property of a set of observations such that they are characteristic of the system from which they are a sample or which they are intended to represent, and thus appropriate to use as the basis for making inferences. A representative sample is one that is free of unacceptably large bias with respect to a particular data quality objective.

Robustness
A criterion used to evaluate the knowledge base uncertainty. It focuses on the predictability of the values and of the results and on the dependency relationships.

Sampling distribution
A probability distribution for a statistic.

Scientific consistency
A criterion used to evaluate the knowledge base uncertainty. It focuses on the maturity of the underlying science and their limitations.

Screening method
A method intended to provide conservative overestimates of exposure and risk using relatively simple and quick calculation methods and with relatively low data input requirements. The purpose of such methods, models or techniques is to eliminate the need for further, more detailed modelling for scenarios that do not cause or contribute to high enough levels of exposure and/or risk to be of potential concern. If a screening method indicates that levels of exposure and/or risk are low, then there should be high confidence that actual exposures and/or risk levels are low. Conversely, if a screening method indicates that estimated exposure and/or risk levels are high, then a more refined method should be applied, since the screening method is intentionally biased. *See* Refined method.

Sensitivity analysis
A study of how the variation in the outputs of a model can be attributed to, qualitatively or quantitatively, different sources of variation in model inputs.

Sensitivity of choices to the analysts' interests
A criterion used to evaluate the subjectivity of choices characteristic of uncertainty.

Statistic
A function of a random sample of data (e.g. mean, standard deviation, distribution parameters).

Statistical uncertainty
Uncertainty associated with randomly drawing samples from a population. Statistics, such as the mean, estimated from a random sample are subject to random fluctuations when estimated repeatedly for independent sets of samples from the same population.

Stochastic process
A process that appears to be random and is not explainable by mechanistic theory. A stochastic process typically refers to variations that can be characterized as a frequency distribution based on observable data but for which there is no useful or practical means to further explain or make predictions based upon the underlying but perhaps unknown cause of the variation. For example, air pollutant concentrations include a stochastic component because of turbulence in the atmosphere that cannot be predicted other than in the form of an average or in the form of a distribution.

Stochastic variability
Sources of heterogeneity of values associated with members of a population that are a fundamental property of a natural system and that as a practical matter cannot be modified, stratified or reduced by any intervention: for example, variation in human susceptibility to

illness for a given dose for which there is no predictive capability to distinguish the response of a specific individual from that of another. Stochastic variability contributes to overall variability for measures of individual risk and for population risk.

Subjective probability distribution
A probability distribution that represents an individual's or group's belief about the range and likelihood of values for a quantity, based upon that person's or group's expert judgement.

Subjectivity of choices
A characteristic of the uncertainty, also called value-ladenness of choices. It is used for qualitative characterization of the source of uncertainty. The subjectivity of choices expresses the influence of the choices made during the exposure assessment, including the influence of situational limitations (e.g. money and time) on choices, the analysts' interests and the subjectivity among peers and stakeholders.

Surrogate data
Substitute data or measurements on one quantity used to estimate analogous or corresponding values of another quantity.

Systematic error
see Bias.

Uncertainty
Uncertainty in risk assessment in the general sense is defined by IPCS (2004) as "imperfect knowledge concerning the present or future state of an organism, system, or (sub)population under consideration". In relation to the specific topic of this monograph, it can be further defined as lack of knowledge regarding the "true" value of a quantity, lack of knowledge regarding which of several alternative model representations best describes a system of interest or lack of knowledge regarding which probability distribution function and its specification should represent a quantity of interest. Uncertainty is related to the epistemic status of an expert community or analysts.

Uncertainty analysis
A methodology that takes into account domain knowledge and its limitations in qualifying or quantifying (or both) the uncertainty in the structure of a scenario, structure of a model, inputs to a model and outputs of a model.

Upper (high-end) bounding
An estimate (e.g. of exposure) that is incurred by an entity or person who is at an upper percentile with respect to the distribution of interindividual variability. A high-end bounding estimate would typically refer to an estimate at or above the 90th percentile of variability. A bounding estimate would typically refer to an estimate that is at least as high as the maximum real-world value and in some cases could be much higher (e.g. a maximally exposed individual).

Variability

Heterogeneity of values over time, space or different members of a population, including stochastic variability and controllable variability. Variability implies real differences among members of that population. For example, different individual persons have different intake and susceptibility. In relation to human exposure assessment, differences over time for a given individual are referred to as intraindividual variability; differences over members of a population at a given time are referred to as interindividual variability.

ANNEX 1: CASE-STUDY—QUALITATIVE UNCERTAINTY ANALYSIS

A1.1 Introduction

This annex aims to illustrate qualitative uncertainty analysis through a case-study that involves estimation of exposure to a persistent, bioaccumulative and lipid-soluble group of chemicals to which humans are exposed mainly through fish consumption, which is referred to here as PBLx. Examples of appropriate communication of the outcome to various target audiences are also considered.

This case-study addresses exposure via ingestion to PBLx in freshwater and marine water fish and shellfish.

Components of uncertainty have been evaluated as Not Applicable (NA), Low, Medium and High in the previously described categories of level of uncertainty, appraisal of the knowledge base and subjectivity of choices (see section 5.1 of the document).

A1.2 Objective

This illustrative practical example of systematic, although qualitative, consideration of uncertainty is based on information included in chapter 3 on sources of uncertainty, in chapter 4 on the tiered approach, in section 5.1 on qualitative uncertainty and in chapter 6 on communication. It includes consensus judgements of uncertainty by a subgroup of the drafting group as a basis for illustration only.

The approach and elements of the characterization of uncertainty are described initially, followed by presentation of the overall outcome and discussion of relevant aspects of communication to various target audiences. A description of the underlying exposure estimation and more detailed information on each of the components are subsequently presented in Appendix 1 to this annex.

A1.3 Sources of uncertainty

Chapter 3 highlighted three basic sources of uncertainty: scenario, model and parameter. Methodology for qualitative characterization of uncertainty presented in section 5.1 focuses on these sources.

Table A1.1 lists the components of uncertainty considered for these three sources in this case-study. For example, for the scenario, eight components have been considered (e.g. target population and exposure event).

Table A1.1: The considered sources of uncertainty.

Sources of uncertainty		
Major	**Detailed**	**Included**
Scenario		Sources/products
		Agent/chemical
		Target population
		Activity
		Chemical emission/release from source
		Exposure pathway
		Exposure event
		Exposure route
Model	Conceptual model	Model assumptions
	Formula	Formula
Parameters	Chemical-specific	Chemical-specific exposure data
	Non-chemical-specific	Non-chemical-specific exposure data

A1.4 Selected tier

Given that identified uncertainties have been characterized qualitatively, this is considered a Tier 1 characterization. At this point, none of the sources has been treated deterministically or probabilistically (i.e. Tier 2 or Tier 3).

Although this case-study does not reflect a Tier 0 level, it does include many of the elements of Tier 0 (i.e. characterization of "level" of uncertainty without analysis of each source), but then moves on to Tier 1 (additionally characterizing individual sources).

A1.5 Characterization and evaluation of uncertainty

Components of sources of uncertainty were systematically considered, in the context of the following characteristics: level of uncertainty, appraisal of the knowledge base and subjectivity of choices, the last two of which include several components (see section 5.1). For appraisal of the knowledge base, these are accuracy, reliability, plausibility, scientific consistency and robustness. For subjectivity of choices, these are choice space, intersubjectivity among peers and stakeholders, influence of situational limitations (e.g. money, tools and time) on choices, sensitivity of choices to the analysts' interests and influence of choices on results.

The overall characterization and evaluation of uncertainty are summarized in Table A1.2. These include presentation of single descriptors where possible and a range of values (e.g. Medium – High) where considerable variation for components precluded aggregation.

Table A1.2: Summary of the Tier 1 uncertainty characterization.

Sources of uncertainty	Characteristics of uncertainty		
	Level of uncertainty	Appraisal of the knowledge base	Subjectivity of choices
Scenario	High	Medium – High	Medium
Model			
Assumptions	Low	Low	Medium – High
Formula	High	High	Low
Parameters			
Chemical-specific exposure data	High	Medium – High	Medium – High
Non-chemical-specific exposure data	High	Low – Medium	Low
Result	High	High	NA

On the basis of this qualitative evaluation, it is clear that the factors impacting exposure are much more complex than those described in the conceptual model. However, simplification was necessitated by limitations of the available data.

Although the level of uncertainty of the model assumptions, structure and details was characterized as "Low" when considered in isolation, the uncertainty of other components (i.e. model extrapolations, chemical-specific exposure data, non-chemical-specific exposure data and exposure assessment result) was considered to be a function primarily of limitations (i.e. simplicity) of the conceptual model.

The uncertainty varies according to the considered sources and characteristics of uncertainty, as shown in Table A1.2.

Tables A1.3 and A1.4 include information on the range of judgements for various components of uncertainty.

Table A1.3: Evaluation of the uncertainties of all sources according to the appraisal of the knowledge base.

Sources of uncertainty	Appraisal of the knowledge base				
	Accuracy	Reliability	Plausibility	Scientific consistency	Robustness
Scenario	High	Medium	High	NA	Medium
Model					
Assumptions	NA	Low	Low	NA	Low
Formula	High	High	High	High	High
Parameters					
Chemical-specific exposure data	Medium	High	Medium	Medium	Medium

Sources of uncertainty	Appraisal of the knowledge base				
	Accuracy	Reliability	Plausibility	Scientific consistency	Robustness
Non-chemical-specific exposure data	Low	Low	Low	NA	Medium
Result	High	High	High	High	High

Table A1.4: Evaluation of the uncertainties of all sources according to the subjectivity of choices.

Sources of uncertainty	Subjectivity of choices				
	Choice space	Intersubjectivity among peers and among stakeholders	Influence of situational limitations on choices	Sensitivity of choices to the analysts' interests	Influence of choices on results
Scenario	Medium	Medium	Medium	Medium	Medium
Model					
Assumptions	Medium	Medium	NA	NA	High
Formula	NA	NA	NA	Low	Low
Parameters					
Chemical-specific exposure data	High	High	NA	Medium	Medium
Non-chemical-specific exposure data	NA	NA	NA	Low	Low
Result	NA	NA	NA	NA	NA

More detailed information on the underlying exposure estimate and a description for each of the judgements are presented in Appendix 1 to this annex.

A1.6 Communication

Examples of appropriate content of communications to various target audiences based on the qualitative uncertainty analysis summarized above are presented below.

A1.6.1 Communication with other scientists

The estimate of the exposure in this example is 0.34 pg/kg body weight per day (see Appendix 1). *Normally, this value is communicated with an estimate of toxicity or together with toxicology-based target values, such as, for example, reference dose (RfD) or acceptable daily intake (ADI).*

It is clear that the factors impacting exposure are much more complex than those described in the conceptual model. However, simplification was necessitated by limitations of the available data.

As part of this exercise, the extent to which the different uncertainties may interact was considered. Therefore, although the level of uncertainty of the model assumptions, structure and details was characterized as "Low" when considered in isolation, the uncertainty of subsequent considerations (i.e. model extrapolations, chemical-specific exposure data, non-chemical-specific exposure data and exposure assessment result) was considered to be a function primarily of limitations (i.e. simplicity) of the conceptual model.

The uncertainty varies according to the considered sources and characteristics of uncertainty, as shown in Table A1.2.

A1.6.2 Communication with risk managers

The exposure of the target population to PBLx has been assessed by a group of internationally recognized experts. The estimate of the exposure is 0.34 pg/kg body weight per day (see Appendix 1). *Normally, this value is communicated with an estimate of toxicity or together with toxicology-based target values, such as, for example, reference dose (RfD) or acceptable daily intake (ADI).*

The estimated exposure is based on some conservative assumptions, but it is not possible to specify the degree of conservatism, owing to the limitations of the available data.

It is clear that the factors impacting exposure are much more complex than those described in the conceptual model. However, simplification was necessitated by limitations of the available data.

As part of this exercise, the extent to which the different uncertainties may interact was considered. Therefore, although the level of uncertainty of the model assumptions, structure and details was characterized as "Low" when considered in isolation, the uncertainty of subsequent considerations (i.e. model extrapolations, chemical-specific exposure data, non-chemical-specific exposure data and exposure assessment result) was considered to be a function primarily of limitations (i.e. simplicity) of the conceptual model.

The uncertainty varies according to the considered sources and characteristics of uncertainty, as shown in Table A1.2.

A1.6.3 Communication with the public

The exposure of the target population to PBLx has been assessed by a group of internationally recognized experts. The estimate of the exposure is 0.34 pg/kg body weight per day. *Normally, this value is communicated with an estimate of toxicity or together with toxicology-based target values, such as, for example, reference dose (RfD) or acceptable daily intake (ADI).*

The estimated exposure is based on some conservative assumptions, but it is not possible to specify the degree of conservatism.

The above statement summarizes the outcomes of the exposure assessment. In order to additionally inform and provide balance for the public, it is important to accompany this statement with information about the risk management conclusions. For example:

Further investigations that clarify the variation over fish species, regional provenance and breeding (e.g. marine versus aquaculture) will be necessary to clarify the extent of variation in exposure.

In the meantime, it is prudent to continue efforts/actions to progressively reduce the levels of exposure to chemicals such as PBLx (1) by means of an overall reduction of environmental pollution and/or (2) by reducing the possible substance uptake through avoiding the consumption of highly contaminated fish species and/or by (3) reducing the frequency of consumption or reduction of meal sizes.

Appendix 1: Background for case-study

Ap1.1 Selected exposure assessment and assumptions

This example is based on calculation of the total average adult daily uptake of unspecified congeners of PBLx per unit body weight from both freshwater and marine water fish and shellfish, according to the following formula:

$$[(2.2 \text{ pg/g} \times 6.0 \text{ g/day} \times 1)/60 \text{ kg}] + [0.51 \text{ pg/g} \times 14.1 \text{ g/day} \times 1)/60 \text{ kg}]$$
$$= 0.22 + 0.12 = 0.34 \text{ pg/kg body weight per day}$$

where:

2.2 pg/g	=	mean concentration of PBLx in *freshwater* fish and shellfish (species-specific ingestion rate weighted averages), from three different studies with different analytical methods and calculation rules, including 12 analyses of pooled samples collected in 1995 from different geographical areas in the United States and analyses of 155 composite samples collected between 1986 and 1988 from five major Canadian cities
0.51 pg/g	=	mean concentration of PBLx in *marine* fish and shellfish (species-specific ingestion rate weighted averages) based on one composite of 13 samples plus five composites from three different studies with different analytical methods and calculation rules, including 12 analyses of pooled samples collected in 1995 from different geographical areas in the United States and analyses of 155 composite samples collected between 1986 and 1988 from five major Canadian cities
6.0 g/day	=	mean daily per capita consumption of *freshwater* fish and shellfish, proposed by USEPA (1997a) for adults based on an extensive database on food consumption patterns
14.1 g/day	=	mean daily per capita consumption of *marine* fish and shellfish proposed by USEPA (1997a) for adults based on an extensive database on food consumption patterns
60 kg	=	mean body weight of the adult population
1	=	assumed absorption following ingestion of 100%

The case-study supposes (1) full agreement about characterization of the issue among stakeholders, (2) well defined objectives of the assessment and (3) adequate communication and understanding by stakeholders and peers of the purpose of the exposure assessment, which is anticipated to be characteristic of circumstances for most regulatory applications.

Ap1.2 Scenario

Eight elements on which the scenario was based were considered in this case-study. Eating patterns may change seasonally, but this element has not been considered. Other aspects that have not been considered include handling and treatment prior to consumption (e.g. supermarket, household cooking, frying). The eight elements are as follows:

1) **Sources:** Two sources are considered: (i) freshwater fish and shellfish; and (ii) marine water fish and shellfish.

2) **Chemical:** PBLx: a persistent, bioaccumulative and lipid-soluble chemical, for which unspecified congeners were considered.

3) **Target population:** Adults randomly selected from a large population.

4) **Activity:** Eating fish and shellfish daily. Even if people do not eat fish and shellfish every day, the study focused on long-term daily averaged consumption.

5) **Chemical emission/release from source:** PBLx in fresh water and marine water are taken up by fish and shellfish and then transferred to humans through their consumption.

6) **Exposure pathway:** Transfer of PBLx from fresh water and marine water into fish and shellfish and then ingested in consumed fish and shellfish. Aquacultured fish are not considered, since PBLx concentrations may vary from those in uncultured varieties. The exposure pathway consists of five steps:
   Step 1:   PBLx in fresh water and marine water.
   Step 2:   PBLx transferred from fresh water and marine water to fish and shellfish through bio-uptake (bioconcentration and/or bioaccumulation).
   Step 3:   Fish and shellfish are transferred from fresh water and marine water to a meal (plate).
   Step 4:   Consumers ingest fish and shellfish.
   Step 5:   PBLx is absorbed in the gastrointestinal tract.

7) **Exposure event:** Consuming freshwater fish, freshwater shellfish, marine fish and marine shellfish.

8) **Exposure route:** Oral exposure.

Characterization of the uncertainties for the eight selected elements of the scenario is presented in Table Ap1.1.

Table Ap1.1: Evaluation of the uncertainties of the scenario.

Level of uncertainty		
High		We cannot trace back to the original (emission) sources. We do not have fully representative data. Methods used in the different studies as a basis for estimation of concentrations are not strictly comparable.
Appraisal of the knowledge base		
Accuracy	High	We have general population data only. We do not have details on variations in consumption patterns. We do not have data on variability within and across fish/shellfish species.
Reliability	Medium	
Plausibility	High	Analytical measurements on fish/shellfish are reliable (uncertainty Low), but there are too few samples and few data on consumption habits (uncertainty High). Methods of analysis and calculation vary within the studies that serve as the basis of concentrations used within the estimates.
Scientific consistency	NA	
Robustness	Medium	
		We are missing description of variation among people, regions and subgroups, including sex. This holds especially for possible high-exposure groups (high fish/shellfish consumption and high PBLx concentration) as well as for non-fish consumers.
		Predictability Low (i.e. not representative).
Subjectivity of choices		
Choice space	Medium	Subjective choices need to be made to focus the assessment (e.g. "seasonal applicability" can be considered and "exposure pathway" can be expanded). Uncertainty for choice space Medium.
Intersubjectivity among peers	Medium	
Influence of situational limitations	Medium	Peers' subjectivity is Medium because we do not know the emission and lack updated information.
Sensitivity of choices	Medium	No funds for new sampling. Limited willingness to fill in the existing data gaps.
Influence of choices on results	Medium	
		Evaluation of the results somewhat depends on the input data and on the stakeholder point of view.
		The choices are bounded by knowledge and by measurement.

Ap1.3 Model

Ap1.3.1 Model assumptions

Estimation of exposure was based on a simple model, which takes into account the four basic components—that is, (i) the concentration of PBLx in fish and shellfish, (ii) the consumption rate of fish and shellfish, (iii) the body weight of adult consumers and (iv) the absorption rate. The absorption rate was set to be 1, which means that 100% is considered to be absorbed in the gastrointestinal tract. This simple model is widely used and accepted as a basic approach to estimate the uptake of chemicals through food consumption. Its level of uncertainty is therefore considered to be Low.

Characterization of the uncertainties for the model is presented in Table Ap1.2.

Table Ap1.2: Evaluation of the uncertainties of the model assumptions.

Level of uncertainty		
Low		The model chosen represents the basic concept and is generally accepted for estimations of uptake if no further differentiation of the source is considered. However, there is some uncertainty associated with lack of detail on numbers of species considered in weighted average concentrations.
Appraisal of the knowledge base		
Accuracy	NA	Because the model is in simple form consistent with existing knowledge, the uncertainty is Low with respect to existing data knowledge.
Reliability	Low	
Plausibility	Low	While simplicity of the model precludes consideration of many influencing factors, input sources and parameters impacting absorption, in view of the limitations of available data, the approach is considered sufficient for a preliminary estimate of average PBLx uptake.
Scientific consistency	NA	
Robustness	Low	
Subjectivity of choices		
Choice space	Medium	Uncertainty for subjectivity is considered Medium because some choices (whether or not consumption is dependent on body weight and sex) are made.
Intersubjectivity among peers	Medium	
Influence of situational limitations	NA	Stakeholders could lobby for different choices (e.g. ages, consumption).
Sensitivity of choices	NA	If a different assumption or approach is selected (e.g. time series versus steady state), the results will change considerably.
Influence of choices on results	High	

Ap1.3.2 Formula

Uptake of PBLx in the general adult population is calculated as a function of mean fish and shellfish consumption rate, mean PBLx concentration in fish and shellfish, mean body weight (BW) and absorption rate (assumed to be 100%):

$$Uptake\ of\ PBLx = \frac{Concentration\ of\ PBLx \times Consumption\ rate \times Absorption\ rate}{BW}$$

It is assumed that there is no change in the concentration of PBLx in the whole fish and shellfish prior to consumption.

Owing to the persistence of PBLx in the body, the exposures from different sources can be summed or added, as is the case for the estimated exposure here, which is based on summed intake from both freshwater and marine fish and shellfish.

Characterization of the uncertainties for the model structure and details is presented in Table Ap1.3.

Table Ap1.3: Evaluation of the uncertainties of the formula.

Level of uncertainty		
High		The formula does not taken into account parameters that may contribute to potential changes in concentrations from live fish and shellfish to cooked meals (see steps of the pathway).
Appraisal of the knowledge base		
Accuracy	High	The knowledge base supports the formula. In other words, the formula fits well the limited existing data.
Reliability	High	
Plausibility	High	However, there is complete lack of knowledge of how cooking influences the concentrations.
Scientific consistency	High	
Robustness	High	
Subjectivity of choices		
Choice space	NA	Uncertainty for subjectivity of choices is Low, although human errors and lack or limitations of review can influence the results.
Intersubjectivity among peers	NA	
Influence of situational limitations	NA	Uncertainty for influence of choices on results is Low because a high level of review/scrutiny is anticipated for any such assessment with regulatory implications.
Sensitivity of choices	Low	
Influence of choices on results	Low	

Ap1.4 Parameters: sample uncertainty

Ap1.4.1 Chemical-specific exposure

Concentration of PBLx in freshwater fish and shellfish	2.2 pg/g
Concentration of PBLx in marine fish and shellfish	0.51 pg/g
Absorption rate of PBLx	100%

Characterization of uncertainties for the chemical-specific exposure data is presented in Table Ap1.4.

Table Ap1.4: Evaluation of the uncertainties of the chemical-specific exposure data.

Level of uncertainty		
High		Estimation of the concentration of PBLx is limited to a single value that is dependent on many parameters (e.g. fish/shellfish species and fish/shellfish size) because of limited sampling.
Appraisal of the knowledge base		
Accuracy	Medium	Uncertainty for the knowledge base is considered Medium because a great deal of information is missing.
Reliability	High	
Plausibility	Medium	Accuracy is limited by the sample size.
Scientific consistency	Medium	Reliability is High because the single value is calculated/transformed.
Robustness	Medium	Uncertainty for plausibility is considered Medium because the single value does not have direct physical correspondence.
		Uncertainty for robustness is considered Medium because of the dependency on the calculation/transformation.
Subjectivity of choices		
Choice space	High	Uncertainty for subjectivity is considered High because of the choice of the calculation. Different stakeholders will have different calculations/transformations.
Intersubjectivity among peers	High	
Influence of situational limitations	NA	Laboratory analysis influences the value.
Sensitivity of choices	Medium	
Influence of choices on results	Medium	

Ap1.4.2 Non-chemical-specific exposure data

Freshwater fish and shellfish consumption rate (dietary ingestion factor)   6.0 g/day
Marine fish and shellfish consumption rate (dietary ingestion factor)   14.1 g/day

The expression of an average fish consumption value derives from nutrition surveys. However, it is not specified if the average value takes into consideration the fish eaters only or the entire population. Thus, the average value is uncertain with respect to its applicability to non-fish eaters. It is also uncertain with respect to its relevance to the overall population or a subpopulation.

The characterization of uncertainties for the non-chemical-specific exposure data is presented in Table Ap1.5.

Table Ap1.5: Evaluation of the uncertainties of the non-chemical-specific exposure data.

Level of uncertainty		
High		The value is single for a multiple-dimension (e.g. sex, season and measurement error) parameter.
Appraisal of the knowledge base		
Accuracy	Low	Uncertainty for the knowledge base is Medium because a great deal of information is missing.
Reliability	Low	
Plausibility	Low	Accurate in the context of what it represents.
Scientific consistency	NA	Reliable in the context of what it represents.
Robustness	Medium	Plausibility is Low because of questionable applicability to different populations.
		Robustness is Medium because of the dependency on body weight, for example.
Subjectivity of choices		
Choice space	NA	Subjectivity is Low.
Intersubjectivity among peers	NA	There may be variability between countries and regions, but the methodology is commonly accepted in a lower-tier assessment.
Influence of situational limitations	NA	
Sensitivity of choices	Low	
Influence of choices on results	Low	

Anthropometric/physiological parameter: body weight   60 kg

The uncertainty of this parameter has not been considered The standard value is questionable because of variation and changes over age and sex. However, within the model, it is not a major source of uncertainty, since additional information on variation in this parameter will not contribute to major changes in the exposure result. A possible 1–2% error in this parameter (used in the denominator of the model) is considered Low in contrast to the major uncertainty sources (e.g. variation in fish-eating habits in the population, mixture of different fish species and degree of contamination associated with regional origin).

Ap1.5 Exposure assessment result

Ap1.5.1 Calculation

The adult daily uptakes of PBLx from freshwater fish and shellfish and from marine water fish and shellfish are estimated to average 0.22 pg/kg body weight per day and 0.12 pg/kg body weight per day, respectively, for a total uptake of 0.34 pg/kg body weight per day.

Ap1.5.2 Output

The uncertainties characterization for the results of the exposure assessment is shown in Table Ap1.6.

Table Ap1.6: Evaluation of the uncertainties of the exposure assessment result.

Level of uncertainty		
High		Uncertainty is considered High because of high uncertainties associated with each of the scenario, input parameters and model extrapolations.
Appraisal of the knowledge base		
Accuracy	High	The knowledge base supports the model structure. However, limitations of available data preclude "validation" of the estimate.
Reliability	High	
Plausibility	High	
Scientific consistency	High	
Robustness	High	
Subjectivity of choices		
Choice space	NA	Subjectivity is NA because it has already been addressed for the components of the calculation.
Intersubjectivity among peers	NA	
Influence of situational limitations	NA	
Sensitivity of choices	NA	
Influence of choices on results	NA	

Part 1: Guidance Document on Characterizing and Communicating Uncertainty in Exposure Assessment

ANNEX 2: CASE-STUDY—QUANTITATIVE UNCERTAINTY ANALYSIS

A2.1 Introduction

This is an example exposure assessment that illustrates quantitative representations of uncertainty and variability at the higher tiers of an exposure assessment. This case-study is based on human exposures to a persistent, bioaccumulative and lipid-soluble compound through fish consumption. This compound is fictional and referred to here as PBLx, but it has properties that correspond to those of known persistent compounds. Specific goals of this case-study are to illustrate (1) the types of uncertainty and variability that arise in exposure assessments, (2) quantitative uncertainty assessment, (3) how distributions are established to represent variability and uncertainty, (4) differences among alternative variance propagation methods, (5) how to distinguish uncertainty from variability and (6) how to communicate the results of an uncertainty analysis.

The overall process of characterizing the exposure scenario along with the magnitude, variability and uncertainty of a specific exposure includes the following steps:

- description of exposure assessment context and question;
- exposure scenario definitions;
- proposed exposure model;
- parameters and data used;
- sensitivity analysis;
- output variance propagation; and
- uncertainty importance evaluation.

Uncertainty analysis and sensitivity analysis are tools that provide insight on how model predictions are affected by data precision. One of the issues in uncertainty analysis that must be confronted is how to rank both individual inputs and groups of inputs according to their contribution to overall uncertainty. In particular, there is a need to distinguish between the relative contribution of true uncertainty versus variability (i.e. heterogeneity), as well as to distinguish model uncertainty from parameter uncertainty. This case-study illustrates methods of uncertainty representation and variance characterization.

A2.2 Methods used in the case-study

The composition of the case-study includes a conceptual model, the modelling approach, construction of input distributions and variance propagation methods. When evaluating uncertainty, it is important to consider how each of these elements contributes to overall uncertainty.

A2.2.1 Conceptual model: the context, the question and scenario development

The goal of the conceptual exposure model is to establish exposure links via exposure pathways to exposure routes and relative magnitude of uptake or intake by different exposure routes (Figure A2.1). Based on the current consensus of the scientific community, exposure is defined in terms of contact with the visible exterior of the person. These contact points include the skin and the openings into the body, such as mouth and nostrils.

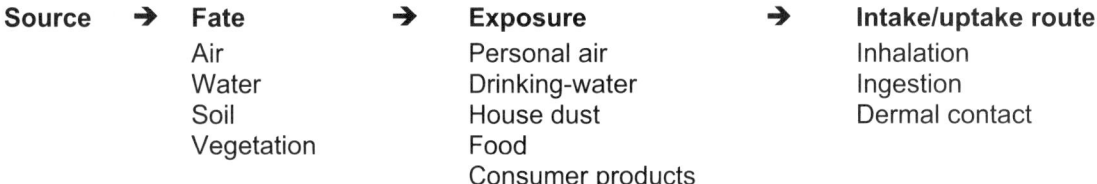

Source	→	Fate	→	Exposure	→	Intake/uptake route
		Air		Personal air		Inhalation
		Water		Drinking-water		Ingestion
		Soil		House dust		Dermal contact
		Vegetation		Food		
				Consumer products		

Figure A2.1: Multimedia, multipathway, multiroute exposure assessment

The conceptual model must address the scenario definition, which includes specification of the pollutant source, environmental transport and transformation, exposure pathways, exposure routes and the amount of chemical taken up through various routes and attributable to specific pathways and sources. The *route of exposure* refers to the way in which an agent enters the receptor during an exposure event. Exposure routes include the inhalation of gases and aerosols, ingestion of fluids and foods, dermal contact with water or soil and dermal uptake of chemicals that contact skin surfaces. Because health impacts of an exposure may vary significantly among the routes of contact, the route of potential uptake is considered a very important attribute of an exposure event. An *environmental pathway* is the course that a chemical or biological agent takes from a source to an exposed individual. This pathway describes a unique mechanism by which an individual or population is exposed to agents originating from a defined location, microenvironment and environmental medium. Exposure scenarios are used to define plausible pathways for human contact.

The general intake model used for the case-study is adapted from a USEPA model. We use this model in the form adopted for generalized multipathway exposure modelling as described in Chapter 6 of IPCS Environmental Health Criteria 214, *Human Exposure Assessment* (IPCS, 2000). In this form, the model expresses the potential average daily intake or potential daily dose, ADD_{pot}, over an averaging time, AT, as

$$ADD_{pot} = \left[\frac{C_i}{C_j}\right] \times \left[\frac{IU_i}{BW}\right] \times \frac{EF \times ED}{AT} \times C_j \qquad [1]$$

where $[C_i/C_j]$ is the intermedia transfer function that relates concentration in medium j to concentration in medium i (e.g. tap water to indoor air); C_i is the contaminant concentration in the exposure medium i; C_j is the contaminant concentration in environmental medium j; IU_i is the intake/uptake factor (per body weight [BW]) for exposure medium i; EF is the exposure frequency (days/year) for this population; ED is the exposure duration (years); and AT is the averaging time for population exposure (days).

A2.2.2 Modelling approach

In the case-study presented below, we apply Equation 1 with the appropriate monitoring data, bioconcentration measurements and human consumption data to make exposure estimates for the exposed population. The model is used to organize and manage information on:

- the magnitude of the source medium concentration: that is, the level of contaminant that is measured or estimated at a release point;
- the contaminant concentration ratio: which defines how much a source medium concentration changes as a result of dilution, transport and intermedia transfers before human contact occurs;
- the level of human contact: which describes (often on a body weight basis) the frequency (days/year) and magnitude (kg/day) of human contact with a potentially contaminated exposure medium;
- the duration of potential contact: relates to the fraction of lifetime, for the population of interest, during which an individual is potentially exposed; and
- the averaging time: the appropriate averaging time is based on the type of health effects under consideration. The averaging time can be the lifetime (as is typical for cancer as an end-point), the exposure duration (as is typical for long-term chronic but non-cancer end-points) or some relatively short time period (as is the case for acute effects).

A2.2.3 Constructing input distributions

The value of information derived from a parameter uncertainty analysis is very much dependent on the care given to the process of constructing the input parameter distributions. One begins the process of constructing a distribution function for a given parameter by assembling values from the literature, from a sampling programme, from experiments and/or from expert knowledge. These values should be consistent with the model and its particular application. The values will vary as a result of measurement error, spatial and temporal variability, extrapolation of data from one situation to another, lack of knowledge, etc. The processes of constructing a distribution from limited and imprecise data can be highly subjective. Because the uncertainty analyst must often apply judgement to this process, there is a need for expertise and wisdom. This process becomes more objective as the number of data for a given parameter increases. However, a large set of data does not necessarily imply the existence of a suitable distribution function.

When constructing input distributions for an uncertainty analysis, it is often useful to present the range of values in terms of a standard probability distribution. It is important that the selected distribution be matched to the range and moments of any available data. In some cases, it is appropriate to simply use the raw data or a custom distribution. Other more commonly used standard probability distributions include the normal distribution, the lognormal distribution, the uniform distribution, the log-uniform distribution and the triangular distribution. For the case-study presented below, we use lognormal distributions.

For any case-study built around Equation 1, we have to consider, for model input, parameters that provide emissions or environmental concentrations, intermedia transfer factors, ingestion (or other intake) rates, body weight, exposure frequency and exposure duration. For our specific case-study below, we are interested in concentrations in surface waters due to deposition from the atmosphere. The relevant intermedia transfer factor is the bioconcentration factor for fish concentration from surface water concentrations. The intake data we need are the magnitude and range of fish ingestion in our exposed population. Because PBLx is a persistent compound that accumulates in fat tissues, we will focus for this case not on exposure frequency and duration but on long-term average daily consumption.

A2.2.4 Variance propagation methods

To carry out the case-study requires the selection of analytical and statistical simulation methods to propagate the parameter variance through to output variance. The methods considered here include analytical variance propagation, factorial design, discrete probability distribution (DPD) arithmetic, unmodified Monte Carlo sampling and a modified Monte Carlo sampling method referred to as Latin hypercube sampling. We illustrate the relative advantages and limitations of these variance propagation methods in our case-study.

For many mathematical operations, including addition, subtraction, multiplication, division, logarithms, exponentials and power relations, there are exact analytical expressions for explicitly propagating input variance and covariance to model predictions of output variance (Bevington, 1969). In analytical variance propagation methods, the mean, variance and covariance matrix of the input distributions are used to determine the mean and variance of the outcome. The following is an example of the exact analytical variance propagation approach. If w is the product of x times y times z, then the equation for the mean or expected value of w, $E(w)$, is:

$$E(w) = E(x) \times E(y) \times E(z) \qquad [2]$$

The variance in w (the standard deviation squared) is given by:

$$\sigma_w^2 = [E(w)]^2 \left\{ \frac{\sigma_x^2}{[E(x)]^2} + \frac{\sigma_y^2}{[E(y)]^2} + \frac{\sigma_z^2}{[E(z)]^2} + \frac{2\sigma_{xy}^2}{[E(x)E(y)]} + \frac{2\sigma_{xz}^2}{[E(x)E(z)]} + \frac{2\sigma_{yz}^2}{[E(y)E(z)]} \right\} \qquad [3]$$

where σ_x^2, σ_y^2, etc. are the variances in x, y, etc. and σ_{xy}^2, σ_{xz}^2, etc., are the covariance of x and y, x and z, etc. The covariance of the population is defined as:

$$\sum_{i=1}^{n} [(x_i - \bar{x})(y_i - \bar{y})] \qquad [4]$$

Bevington (1969) lists variance propagation solutions like the one above for several mathematical operations.

In a factorial design, we represent each model input by a small number (n) of values that characterize the range of the inputs. It is typical that n is 2 (High, Low) or 3 (High, Medium, Low), and the estimates of High and Low represent a range predefined by confidence limits. If there are m model inputs, then a factorial design requires n^m calculations of an outcome. For example, a model with three inputs represented by three levels (High, Medium, Low) has 27 outcomes—HHH, HHM, HMH, HMM, MHH, MHM, MMM, … LLL. In this case, the outcome variance can be estimated from the variance in the 27 predicted outcomes. Correlation effects cannot be characterized using simple factorial design.

DPD arithmetic is a method for replacing continuous distributions with simple discrete distributions that approximate the confidence intervals and the moments (e.g. mean and variance) of the distribution being approximated. The penalty for this simplification is some loss of information about the shape of the inputs and the sources of variance. In a DPD approach, the "high" value is selected to represent the mean of a specified segment (e.g. upper 33%) of a distribution. This condenses the number of discrete values used to represent each factorial combination. Operationally, the DPD approach works like the factorial design. The major difference is in the level of effort used to select a small set of values to represent an input distribution. In the factorial design, a high value represents an upper bound of the distribution, the middle value, the centre, etc. In addition, DPD differs from the factorial method by allowing, with some effort, inclusion of some correlations among the inputs (Morgan & Henrion, 1990).

In an unmodified Monte Carlo method, simple random sampling is used to select each member of the m-tuple set. Each of the input parameters for a model is represented by a probability density function that defines both the range of values that the input parameters can have and the probability that the parameters are within any subinterval of that range. In order to carry out a Monte Carlo sampling analysis, each input is represented by a cumulative distribution function (CDF) in which there is a one-to-one correspondence between a probability and values. A random number generator is used to select probability in the range of 0–1. This probability is then used to select a corresponding parameter value.

In contrast to unmodified Monte Carlo sampling, Latin hypercube sampling uses "stratified" random sampling to select each member of an m-tuple set. Whereas simple random sampling uses chance to evenly select values in the range of an input parameter, Latin hypercube sampling places restrictions on possible unevenness (Iman & Shortencarier, 1984). To generate an m-tuple set using Latin hypercube sampling, each input distribution is divided into k intervals of equal probability. From these intervals, random variables may be selected in two ways. In "normal" Latin hypercube sampling, values are chosen randomly from each probability interval. Alternatively, a midpoint method, similar to the discrete and factorial designs, uses the median of each interval as inputs (Morgan & Henrion, 1990). This selection process is repeated for all the probabilistic inputs. In this way, sample scenario inputs converge more rapidly towards the true outcome moments.

A2.3 Case-study: PBLx exposure from fish ingestion

As a specific case-study, we constructed information on a chemical designated as PBLx. This compound is persistent both in the ambient environment and in human tissues. It is also bioaccumulative and lipid soluble. PBLx is a dioxin-like compound. However, it should be noted that this example does not reflect WHO recommendations for dioxin exposure assessment. We consider long-term historical releases of PBLx to the atmosphere over large regions with resulting global deposition to both ocean and surface waters. Measurements reveal that concentrations of PBLx in ocean and surface waters are similar. In both ocean and surface waters, this compound is transferred to the tissues of fish that are consumed by humans. There are laboratory measurements of PBLx bioconcentration or biotransfer factors (BCFs), but these measurements do not provide sufficient information to establish different PBLx BCF values in ocean and surface waters. So we must assume that these measurements reflect the BCF that would be observed in either ocean or surface water. We also have information on fish consumption that can be used to assess human contact. Because our water concentration data and BCF measurements are not specific to either ocean or freshwater systems, we do not attempt to distinguish consumption according to ocean or freshwater sources.

A2.3.1 Elements of the exposure assessment: context and question

In this case-study, the issue of concern is the extensive exposure of human populations to PBLx, which is a persistent pollutant with multimedia and multipathway exposure potential. For PBLx, exposures occur primarily through food pathways. Here we focus on fish ingestion exposures from PBLx emissions to air that are deposited on ocean and fresh waters and accumulated in both ocean and freshwater fish. This situation focuses attention on three key pieces of information—concentration in water, biotransfer to fish and human consumption of fish.

A2.3.2 Scenario definition

PBLx exposure through fish ingestion represents a case in which highly variable and uncertain data must be characterized. The exposure route involves the ingestion of fish contaminated by PBLx and incorporates the variability/uncertainty in water concentrations, a fish BCF and fish intake to define the variance in the distribution of likely human intake of PBLx.

A2.3.3 Model selection

In order to illustrate the use of the variance propagation methods described above, we have selected for the case-study a simple three-input exposure model. The three inputs for this model include water concentration, fish BCF and fish consumption rates. The model output is dose expressed in micrograms per day averaged over a one-year exposure period. This model has the form:

$$\text{Intake (µg/day)} = \text{Water concentration (ng/l)} \times \text{BCF (l/kg)} \times \text{Fish ingestion (kg/day)} \times 10^{-3} \text{ µg/ng} \qquad [5]$$

where the water concentration (in ng/l) is the measured concentration of PBLx in both ocean and surface waters, BCF is the bioconcentration factor relating PBLx concentration in fish tissue (ng/kg) to PBLx concentration in water (ng/l) and fish ingestion (in kg/day) refers to the yearly-averaged daily human intake of fish from either ocean or surface water bodies. Because our period of assessment is one year, the exposure duration and averaging time are assumed equal. Moreover, because we are interested in long-term cumulative intake during this one-year period, we assume the exposure frequency to be 365 days/year.

A2.3.4 Parameter values and data

The data needed for this exposure assessment include surface water concentrations based on limited monitoring data from fresh and ocean water, laboratory-scale BCF experiments and activity patterns (variation in long-term average fish consumption). We also have biomonitoring data derived from limited geographical, temporal and population subgroup coverage.

Table A2.1 summarizes the surface water concentration data available for making an estimate of the magnitude and range of concentrations of PBLx in fresh and ocean waters. Figure A2.2 provides a probability plot in which the cumulative distribution as reflected in the Z score is plotted against water concentrations for both surface and ocean waters.

Table A2.1: Surface water concentration data for PBLx.

Chemical	Total number of samples	Limit of detection (LOD) (ng/l)	Number of samples >LOD	Concentration range (ng/l)	Median concentration (ng/l)	Surface water type
PBLx	16	9	6	<LOD to 150	15.5	Fresh water
PBLx	35	9	14	<LOD to 200	20	Ocean

The value of a quantitative uncertainty analysis depends on the care given to the process of constructing probability distributions. The process of constructing a distribution from limited and imprecise data can be highly subjective. This process becomes more objective as the number of data for a given parameter increases. However, a large set of data does not necessarily imply the existence of a suitable distribution function.

Based on the data summarized in Table A2.1 and Figure A2.2, we are required to make assumptions to complete our uncertainty analysis. The number of positive samples, within the limit of detection, is low for both ocean and surface waters. In order to develop a probability distribution as well as moments (mean, standard deviation) for our analysis, we must consider some method to represent observations below the LOD. We construct a cumulative probability plot under the assumption that values below the LOD provide an estimate of the cumulative number of sample values above the LOD. This allows us to combine the ocean and freshwater samples so as to construct a probability distribution to fit these observations. This process is illustrated in Figure A2.2.

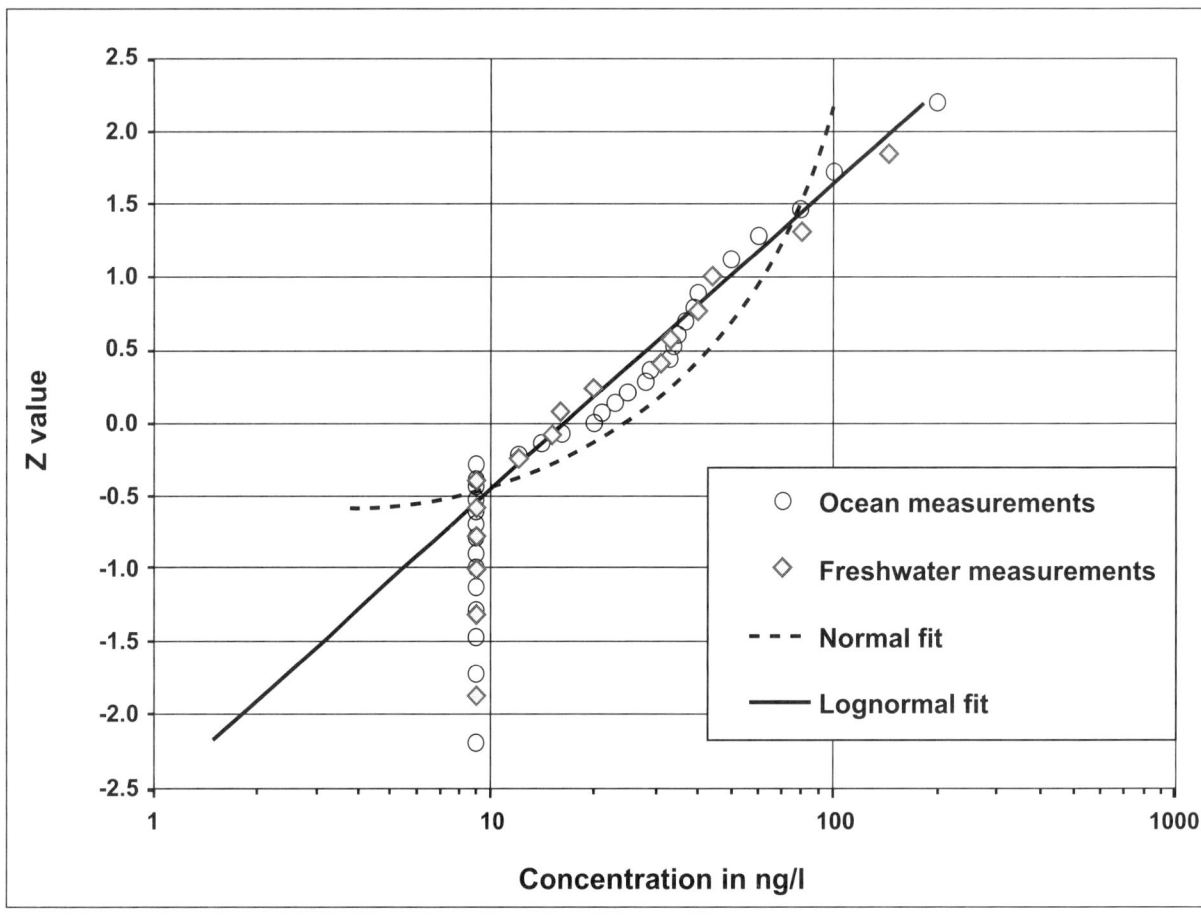

Figure A2.2: Probability plot showing the distribution of water sample concentration data in oceans and fresh water and the lognormal distribution used to represent these concentration data

When constructing input distributions for an uncertainty analysis, it is often useful to present the range of values in terms of a standard probability distribution. It is important that the selected distribution be matched to the range and moments of any available data. Commonly used standard probability distributions include the normal distribution, lognormal distribution, uniform distribution, log-uniform distribution, triangular distribution, beta distribution, gamma distribution and logistic distribution. Modellers use various subjective, graphical and statistical methods to select an appropriate distribution to represent a set of input values. In the probability plot provided in Figure A2.2, we can graphically compare how well the standard normal or standard lognormal distribution fits the set of concentration observations. Here we see a much better fit of the observations with a lognormal distribution. Statistical goodness-of-fit tests confirm that the lognormal distribution best fits these data.

In Table A2.2, we summarize the statistical moments—arithmetic mean and standard deviation (SD), coefficient of variation (CV), and geometric mean (GM) and geometric standard deviation (GSD)—of the lognormal distribution used to represent the combined distribution of ocean and freshwater samples. We also provide the variation of fish ingestion for the case-study. For this, we use fish ingestion rates taken from Ruffle et al. (1994), who examined variation of fish ingestion by adults in the United States. They used a lognormal distribution to represent this fish ingestion variation. The statistical moments of this distribution are summarized in Table A2.2.

Table A2.2: Statistical moments for model parameters in each scenario.

Input parameters	Mean	SD	CV	Geometric mean	GSD
Water concentration (ng/l)	30.9	37.1	1.20	16.4	3.0
BCF (l/kg)	12 700	13 500	1.07	7700	3.1
Human ingestion of fish (kg/day)	0.000 34	0.000 057	0.17	0.000 33	1.2

Fish BCF distributions for PBLx were constructed from data collected at six different laboratories where experimental measurements were carried out on multiple fish species. The range of measured BCF values is displayed in Table A2.3, along with information on the fish species used and laboratory where the experiments were carried out.

The data in Table A2.3 were used to construct a lognormal distribution of variation in these BCF values. We consider this variation to represent the uncertainty about what BCF value to apply to the surface water concentrations to translate the water concentration to a fish concentration. In Figure A2.3, we plot the cumulative number of measurements expressed as Z score against the range of BCF values. We then draw a straight line through these points to obtain the lognormal distribution that best fits this range of BCF values. The statistical moments of this line are summarized in Table A2.2.

Table A2.3: BCF data for PBLx in fish.

Log(BCF)	Fish type	Source
3.1	Fathead minnow (*Pimephales promelas*)	Laboratory 1
3.25	Guppy (*Poecilia reticulata*)	Laboratory 2
3.31	Rainbow trout (*Oncorhynchus mykiss*)	Laboratory 3
3.4	Rainbow trout (*Oncorhynchus mykiss*)	Laboratory 3
3.55	Channel catfish (*Ictalurus punctatus*)	Laboratory 1
3.6	Fathead minnow (*Pimephales promelas*)	Laboratory 3
3.85	Fathead minnow (*Pimephales promelas*)	Laboratory 3
3.9	Mosquito fish (*Gambusia affinis*)	Laboratory 4
3.95	Fathead minnow (*Pimephales promelas*)	Laboratory 5
4.11	Rainbow trout (*Oncorhynchus mykiss*)	Laboratory 5
4.2	Guppy (*Poecilia reticulata*)	Laboratory 5
4.3	Rainbow trout (*Oncorhynchus mykiss*)	Laboratory 6
4.43	No specific species described	Laboratory 6
4.5	Rainbow trout (*Oncorhynchus mykiss*)	Laboratory 6
4.7	Goldfish (*Carassius auratus*)	Laboratory 6

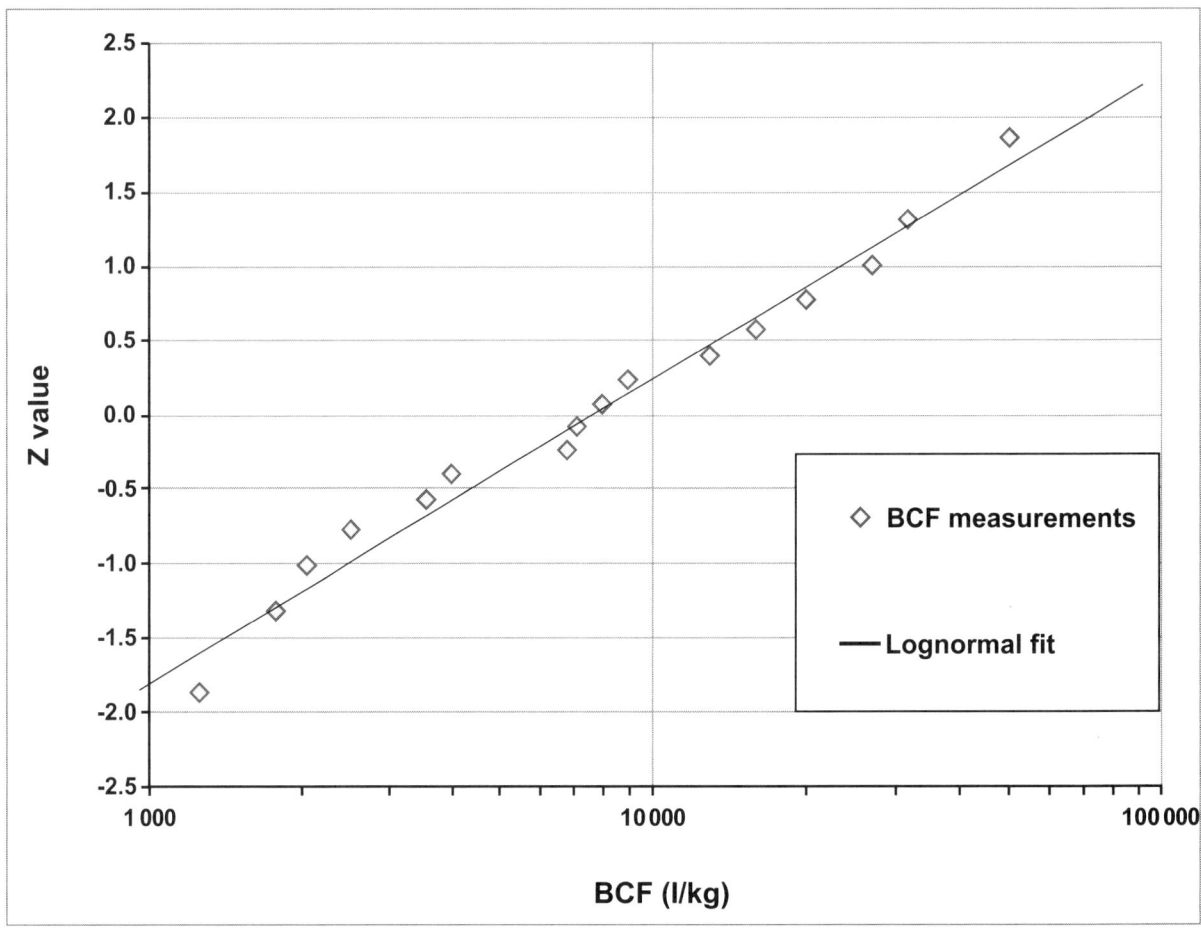

Figure A2.3: Probability plot showing the distribution of measured BCF values and the lognormal distribution used to represent the variation in these measured values

A2.3.5 Worst-case scenario

In order to contrast an uncertainty analysis with what is often common practice in risk assessment, we consider first the worst-case scenario. For the fish intake exposure pathway in our case-study, the worst case would be the person who consumes the most fish, eating fish with the highest observed BCF taken from a water supply with the highest observed concentration of PBLx. The highest observed concentration of PBLx is 200 ng/l. The highest observed log BCF in the reported experiments is 4.7, with a corresponding BCF of 50 100. We then consider the highest continuous fish consumption as the 95% upper confidence limit on fish consumption in the reported data, a value of 0.000 51 kg/day. Combining these values in our exposure equation (Equation 5) gives a worst-case scenario intake of 5.5 µg of PBLx per day.

A2.3.6 Variance propagation

In order to determine variation in PBLx intake resulting from the variance (due to uncertainty and variability) in the parameters used to describe the source-to-dose model, we first use the analytical method to propagate model variance in Equation 2 using moments taken directly from Table A2.2. We then make use of the data in Table A2.2 to set up factorial design, DPD, Monte Carlo sampling and Latin hypercube sampling simulations. In the factorial design approach, we used three values to represent the distribution of each of three inputs, yielding 27 combinations of "Low", "Medium" and "High". As prescribed by the method, "Medium" describes the median of the parameter value range, and "High" and "Low" represent the observed upper and lower extremes. In the case of fish intake, however, original data were not available. "High" and "Low" values were set to represent values at three standard deviations from the means. The high, medium and low values used in the factorial design analysis are listed in Table A2.4.

Table A2.4: Factorial design method values.

	Low	Medium	High
Water concentration (ng/l)	5	20	200
BCF (l/kg)	1300	7500	50 000
Fish consumption (kg/day)	0.000 17	0.000 34	0.000 51

For the DPD method, as for the factorial design example above, we used three input variables and a "High", "Medium" and "Low" value to represent each input distribution. The values used to represent these ranges are listed in Table A2.5. In the DPD case, the "High" and "Low" values were calculated as the median values of the upper and lower 33rd percentiles of the lognormal distributions used to represent the variance of the input parameters. The "Medium" value was set at the median value of each input distribution.

Table A2.5: DPD method input values.

	Low	Medium	High
Water concentration (ng/l)	5.4	20	50
BCF (l/kg)	2500	7500	24 000
Fish consumption (kg/day)	0.000 28	0.000 34	0.000 39

A2.3.7 Variance propagation with uncertainty and variability combined

Model variance was propagated using the factorial, DPD, Monte Carlo and Latin hypercube sampling (LHS) methods. Table A2.6 provides a summary comparison of the outputs—the arithmetic mean, arithmetic standard deviation, coefficient of variation (CV), geometric mean (GM), geometric standard deviation (GSD), 5th percentile and 95th percentile outcomes—from each method.

Table A2.6: Selected statistics of the PBLx intake distribution obtained from different model variance propagation methods.

	Analytical	Monte Carlo (2000)	LHS (200)	DPD	Factorial design
Mean (μg/day)	0.13	0.13	0.14	0.081	0.5
Standard deviation (SD)	0.36	0.28	0.29	0.1	1.2
Coefficient of variation (CV)	2.8	2.2	2.2	1.2	2.4
Geometric mean (GM) (μg/day)	0.043	0.042	0.042	0.041	0.065
GSD	4.4	4.7	5.4	3.5	9.3
5th percentile (μg/day)	0.0037	0.0034	0.0021	0.0041	0.0015
95th percentile (μg/day)	0.49	0.52	0.54	0.38	2.2

The differences in estimation of these moments for each scenario are graphically illustrated in Figures A2.4, A2.5 and A2.6, where the CDFs obtained from each numerical variance propagation method are compared with the analytical results. The results of the analytical method are assumed to represent the true moments of the model output and, therefore, the true CDF. Mean and standard deviation of ln(x) are used in plotting the analytical CDF. The equations for the transformation from arithmetic moments to the moments of ln(x) are as follows:

$$\mu_1 = \text{mean of } \ln(x) = \ln \mu - 0.5\,(\sigma_1^2) \tag{6}$$

$$\sigma_1 = \text{SD of } \ln(x) = \sqrt{\ln\!\left(1 + \frac{\sigma^2}{\mu^2}\right)} \tag{7}$$

Figure A2.4 compares the CDFs for intake obtained from factorial design and DPD methods with the exact analytical solution for the CDF of intake. The 27 data points from the DPD and factorial methods were used to plot the empirical CDF shown in Figure A2.4. Figure A2.5 compares the CDF for intake obtained from 2000 Monte Carlo simulations with the exact analytical solution for the CDF of intake. Figure A2.6 compares the CDF obtained from 200 Latin hypercube sampling Monte Carlo simulations with the exact analytical solution for the CDF of intake. The Monte Carlo and Latin hypercube sampling empirical CDFs were plotted using all simulation outcomes.

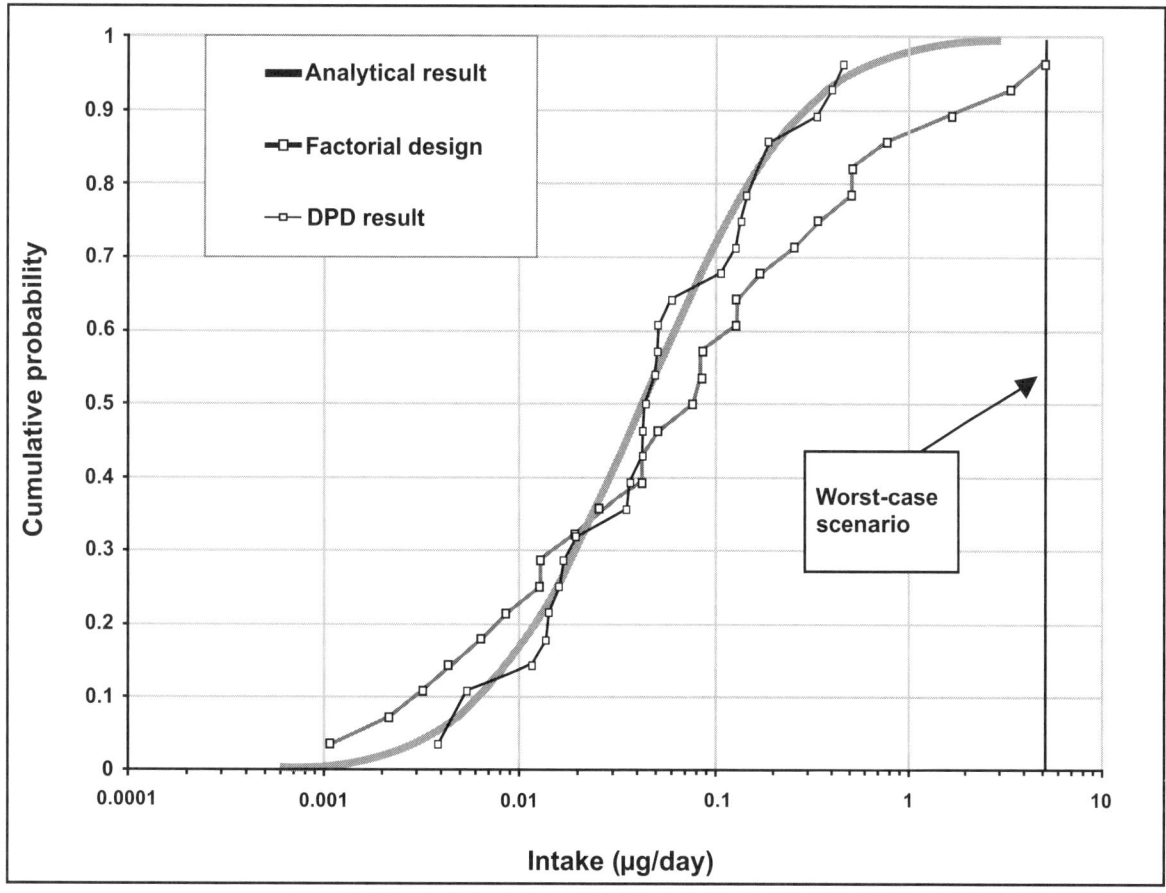

Figure A2.4: Comparison of the CDFs for intake obtained from factorial design and DPD methods with the exact analytical solution for the CDF of intake and with the worst-case scenario

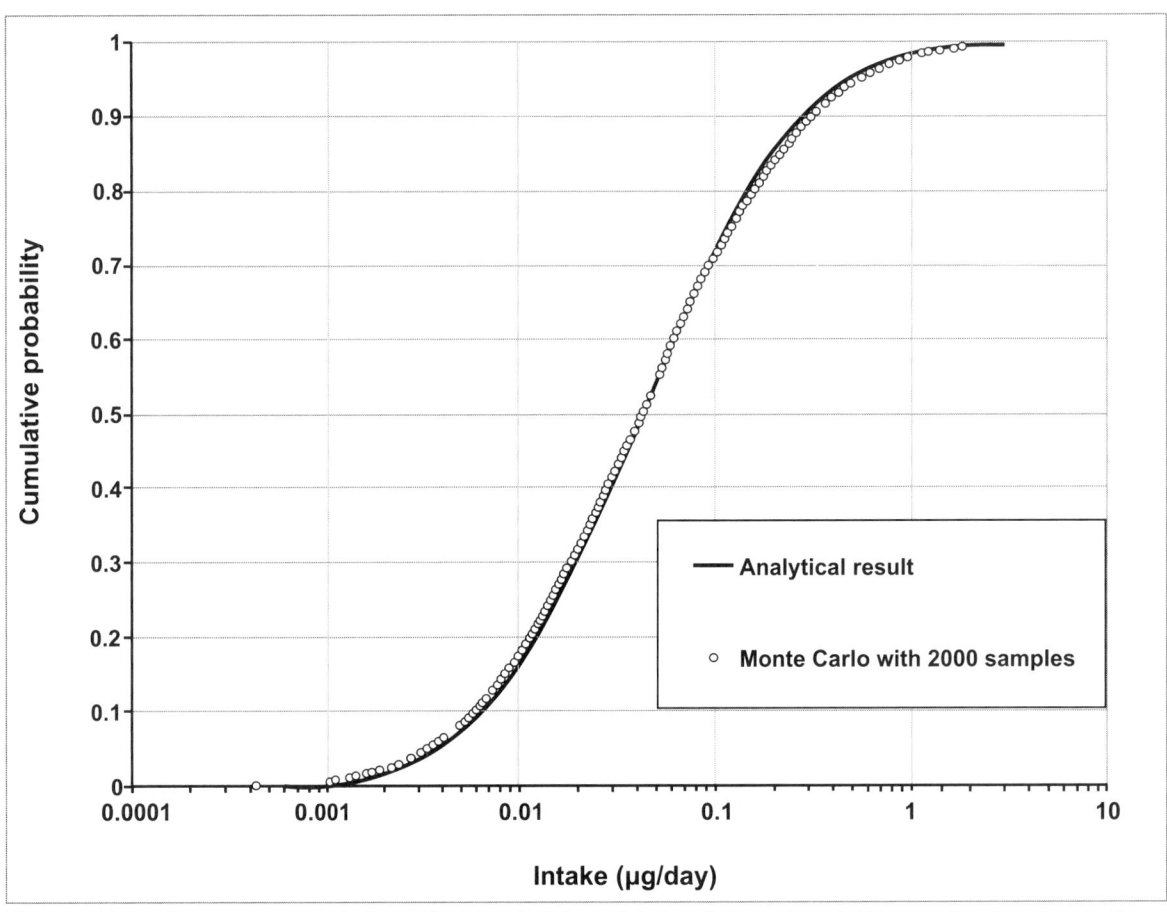

Figure A2.5: Comparison of the CDF for intake obtained from 2000 Monte Carlo simulations with the CDF from the exact analytical solution for intake

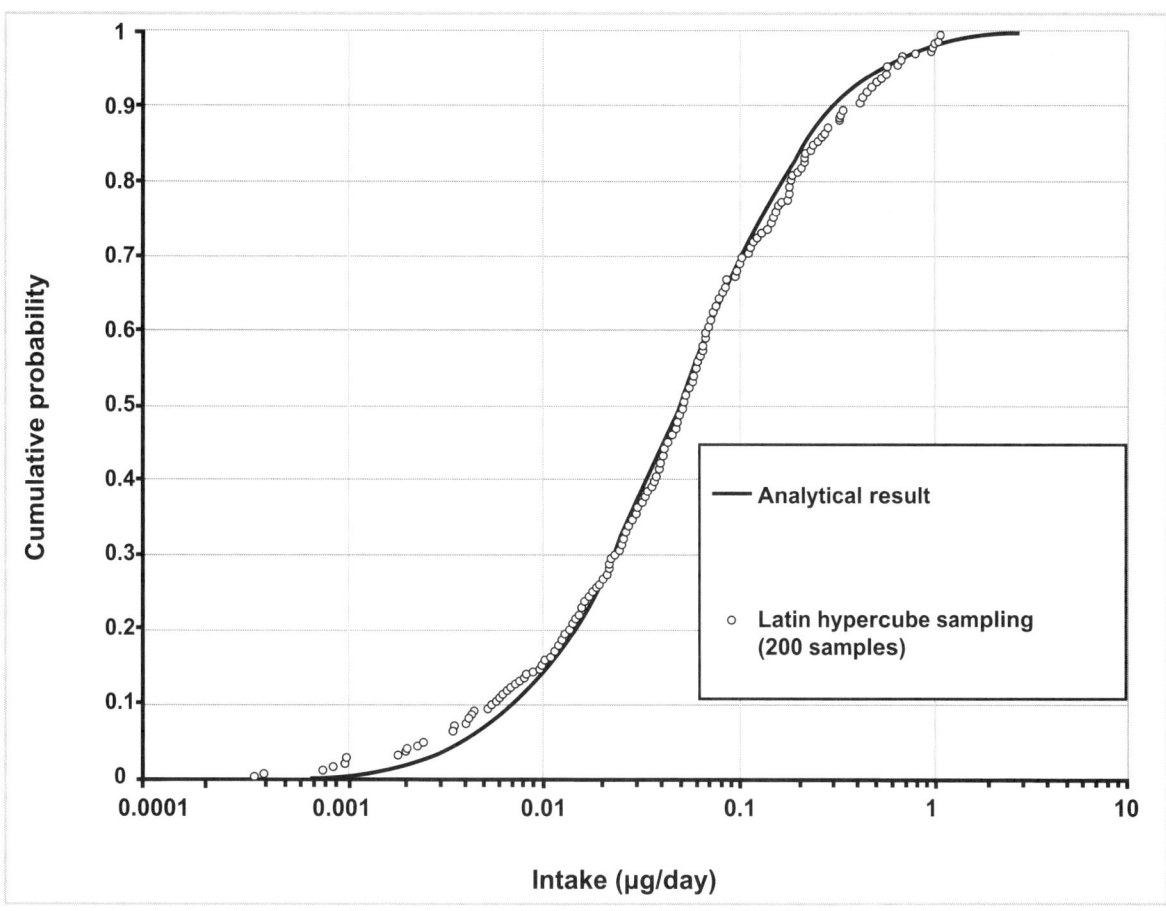

Figure A2.6: Comparison of the CDF for intake obtained from 200 Latin hypercube sampling Monte Carlo simulations with the CDF from the exact analytical solution for intake

From Table A2.6 and Figures A2.5 and A2.6, we see that Monte Carlo and Latin hypercube sampling provide very good agreement both with respect to finding the appropriate moments of the outcome distribution and with respect to the graphical fit. In contrast, the DPD and the factorial design methods are effective only in capturing preliminary estimates of the mid-range values and first estimates of the spread of the outcome distributions. The factorial design, because the highest and lowest observed values are typically used to represent the upper and lower segments of the distribution, provides a reasonable estimate of the distributional midpoint and range, but overstates the variance, coefficient of variation and mean considerably. The DPD, while similar in approach to the factorial design, employs the true moments of each third of the distribution. This results in a more accurate representation of the linear range of the CDF (Figure A2.4). However, even for DPD, the tails tend to deviate from those observed in the analytical, Latin hypercube sampling or Monte Carlo approaches. This is due, primarily, to the limited number of segments used to represent input distributions and contributes to the understatement of variance. Theoretically, calculation using more quantiles in either the DPD or factorial method would improve the output representation; however, computational complexity increases geometrically with each additional segment used to represent inputs for these methods. In contrast to the approximate analytical solutions (factorial design and DPD), the Monte Carlo and Latin hypercube sampling both tend to track the "true" (analytical) outcome distribution quite well.

Comparing all of the distribution results to the "worst-case" scenario gives insight on the problem of using a worst-case scenario. In comparison with the results in Table A2.6 and Figures A2.4 through A2.6, the worst-case intake (5 µg/day) is an order of magnitude higher than the 95% upper confidence limit value of intake obtained from the analytical, Monte Carlo, Latin hypercube sampling and DPD arithmetic methods. The worst-case result is even significantly higher than the upper 95th percentile outcome from the factorial design—an approach shown above to significantly overestimate the upper ranges of exposure relative to the analytical (exact) variance propagation method.

This relatively simple model illustrates the viability of the straightforward analytical analysis. Most models, unfortunately, involve many more input variables and proportionally more complex formulae to propagate variance. Fortunately, the Latin hypercube sampling and Monte Carlo methods simplify complex model variance analysis.

A2.3.8 Variance propagation with uncertainty and variability separated

So far in the case-study, we have focused on variance propagation methods and have not made an effort to distinguish between the relative contributions to overall variance from uncertainty and variability. In the examples above, the cumulative distributions presented in figures all reflect overall variance that includes the combined contributions from both uncertainty and variability. So our last step is to illustrate a two-dimensional analysis in which we distinguish and display separate contributions from uncertainty and variability. We begin this analysis by going back to our inputs and assessing the relative contributions from uncertainty and variability.

First we consider the concentration, C_w, of PBLx in surface water. Previously in this annex, we showed that the observed ocean and freshwater data for concentration could be fit to a lognormal distribution. However, we recognized that in the context of the exposed population, there is variability in this parameter attributable to spatial and seasonal variability as well as uncertainty due to measurement error and due to the representativeness of the sample size. Thus, the standard deviation observed in Figure A2.2 includes variance due to both variability and uncertainty. We assume now that we have conducted an evaluation that indicates that only 30% of the observed variance is due to variability and the remaining 70% of the observed variance is attributable to uncertainty. This evaluation is carried out by Monte Carlo simulation of the experimental method. That is, we consider how much variance due to measurement error and due to small sample size we would observe for any set of observations of the same concentration. We then simulate a set of observations that have a range of values for samples that were at the same concentration. We then use Monte Carlo sampling from the lognormal distribution shown in Figure A2.2 to obtain a second set with the same number of observations. Using rank correlation to compare the spread of observations from a set of samples all the same concentration with a set of samples selected from the distribution in Figure A2.2, we find that 30% of the full variance is explained by variation in observing a single value. Because the lognormal distribution in Figure A2.2 has both true variability and uncertainty, the concentration data can be represented by a family of distributions with a variance having a geometric standard deviation of 1.64 due to variability. These curves have a location range that spans a range with a geometric standard deviation of 2.51. This is illustrated in Figure A2.7. Here we see that when uncertainty is separated from variability, the result is a range of curves reflecting variability at different confidence levels with respect to uncertainty. In this example, we make all curves go through the same median point so that all curves of variability have the same geometric mean. With this approach, we impose uncertainty on the variance of concentration but not on the geometric mean. It is more typical to use a set of curves that have different means and variance to better map out uncertainty about a range of curves that can fit these observations.

Next we consider the bioconcentration factor, BCF, of PBLx. Previously in this annex, we used results from a series of experiments to develop for BCF a probability distribution that includes both variability and uncertainty. Again, an assumed evaluation of the data and measurements indicates that only 40% of the observed variance is due to variability and the remaining 60% of the observed variance is attributable to uncertainty. So the concentration data consist of a family of distributions with a variance having a geometric standard deviation of 1.93 due to variability. These curves have a location range that spans a range with a geometric standard deviation of 2.37.

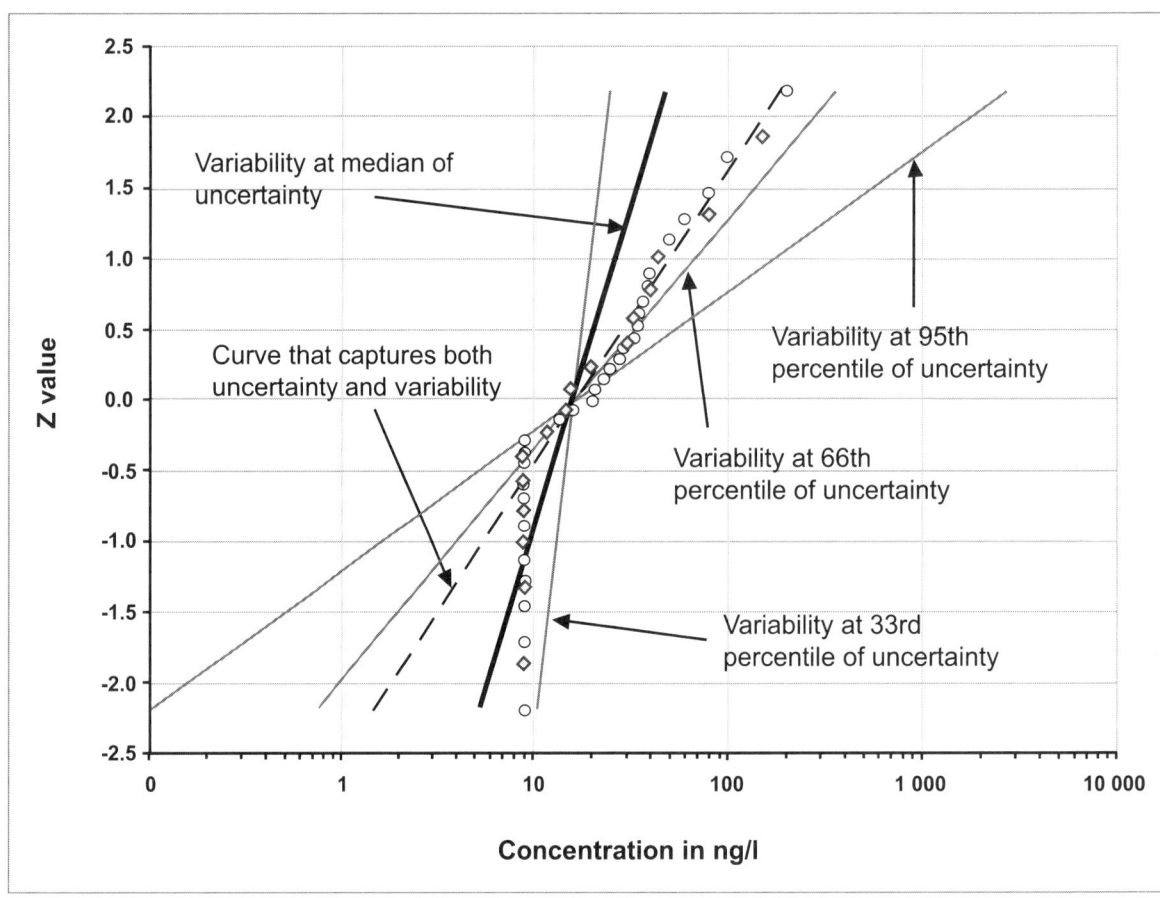

Figure A2.7: The family of curves reflecting variability at different confidence intervals with respect to uncertainty in the data used to assess the variance in surface water concentration for PBLx

Finally, we consider the data on fish ingestion. Here we note that essentially all of the variance in the probability distribution used to represent observations on fish consumption reflects variability. So in this case, the curve reflecting both variability and uncertainty is assumed to be the same as the curve reflecting variability.

We now repeat our Monte Carlo assessment using a nested approach that separates out uncertainty and variability. For both C_w and BCF, we simulate uncertainty by selecting a factor from a lognormal distribution with a geometric mean of 1 and a geometric standard deviation of 2.51 and 2.37, respectively. This factor is applied to each estimate of intake that is obtained from Monte Carlo sampling from the distributions of variability only for C_w, BCF and fish ingestion. This process generates one curve of variability for each outer loop with a selected geometric standard deviation for uncertainty in C_w and BCF. The results of this process are illustrated in Figure A2.8, which shows examples of the curves that can be plotted from this type of nested Monte Carlo analysis.

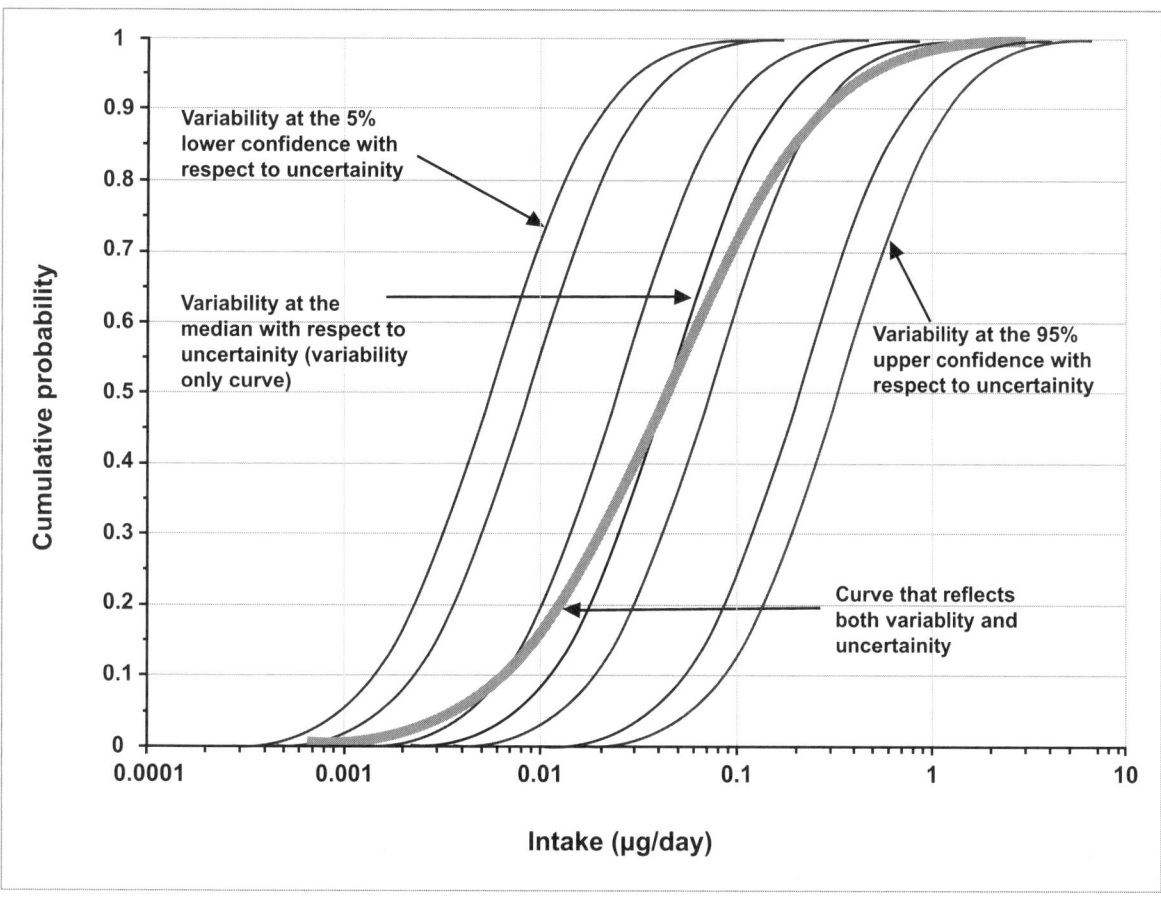

Figure A2.8: Examples of the curves that can be plotted from this type of nested Monte Carlo analysis

Figure A2.8 illustrates the results of a nested, two-dimensional quantitative uncertainty assessment. In Figures A2.4 through A2.6, we presented the results of an uncertainty assessment by allowing the variance in each parameter to be represented by a single distribution with a range and standard deviation that represent both variability (heterogeneity) and true uncertainty. Now we recognize that, for each parameter, some of the observed variance is due to uncertainty and some is due to variability, and we separate out these components. Figure A2.8 shows the results of making this separation. For reference, the thick grey line shows a cumulative distribution of intake when uncertainty and variability in each parameter are combined—as was obtained in Figures A2.4 through A2.6. The other curves are examples of cumulative distributions of variability that result at different levels of uncertainty. When we make 1000 outer loop (uncertainty) calculations by Monte Carlo sampling from the distributions of uncertainty for each parameter, we obtain 1000 cumulative distributions for variability. For each of these outer loop simulations, we fix the selected uncertainty parameters and then run a second Monte Carlo assessment by randomly selecting from distributions of variability. The resulting set of 1000 cumulative distribution curves reflects both uncertainty and variability. We can order these curves from left to right based on the median value of intake obtained in each curve as illustrated in Figure A2.8 with a small subset of these curves. From this set of 1000 curves, the 50th curve in the set would be the curve corresponding to the 5% lower confidence bound value of intake with respect to uncertainty at any given percentile of variability. The 500th curve in the set would be the curve corresponding to the median intake value with respect to uncertainty at any given percentile of variability. The 950th curve in the set would be the curve corresponding to the 95% upper confidence bound with respect to uncertainty at any given percentile of variability. These select curves are identified for our case-study in Figure A2.8.

A2.4 Summary of the case-study

This case-study addresses the problem of defining, characterizing and propagating uncertainty in an exposure model. Uncertainty analysis is used to assess the impact of data precision on model predictions. A common complaint associated with "worst-case" approaches to risk assessment is that the use of highly conservative values for each input variable results in significant overestimation of actual risk and/or exposure factors.

Characterization and propagation of variance for input parameters do two things. First, they give the decision-maker a more realistic view of how estimates can spread, given what is known about the inputs. Secondly, instead of a point value, variance propagation quantifies output certainty, allowing assessment of its accuracy and usefulness. In this case-study, we illustrate how different variance propagation methods make possible different levels of evaluation, depending on the information available, the complexity of the model and the accuracy needed. The case-study illustrates a strategy for evaluating the sources of uncertainty in predictive exposure assessments. The methods and examples presented make clear that risk managers should be aware of the uncertainty in risk estimates and include this awareness in their decisions and their communications of risk to the public. As illustrated in the case-study, one of the issues in uncertainty analysis that must be addressed is the need to distinguish between the relative contributions of true uncertainty and variability (i.e. heterogeneity).

PART 2:
HALLMARKS OF DATA QUALITY IN CHEMICAL EXPOSURE ASSESSMENT

PREPARATION OF THE DOCUMENT

This document was developed in accordance with World Health Organization (WHO)/International Programme on Chemical Safety (IPCS) processes, involving meetings of experts to develop a draft document, public review and peer review, followed by expert discussions to consider the comments received and finalize the document. In developing the draft document, the experts identified and considered a range of publications on the topic, including national guidance (which was available only from the United States of America [USA]). The stages and experts involved are listed below.

Preparation of public review draft

The public review draft of this document was developed in two stages: an IPCS Data Quality Drafting Group prepared the draft text, then an IPCS Harmonization Group provided additional input.

Members of the IPCS Data Quality Drafting Group

Dr Nancy B. Beck
Toxicologist/Risk Assessor, Office of Information and Regulatory Affairs, Office of Management and Budget, Executive Office of the President, Washington, DC, USA

Dr William C. Griffith *(Chair)*
Associate Director, Institute for Risk Analysis and Risk Communication, Department of Environmental and Occupational Health Sciences, University of Washington, Seattle, WA, USA

Dr Chris Money
Industrial Hygiene Advisor – Europe, Exxon Mobil Petroleum & Chemical, Machelen, Belgium

Dr Sumol Pavittranon
Office of Risk Assessment, National Institute of Health, Ministry of Public Health, Nonthaburi, Thailand

Secretariat

Ms Carolyn Vickers
International Programme on Chemical Safety, World Health Organization, Geneva, Switzerland

Members of the IPCS Harmonization Group

Dr Andy Hart
Risk Analysis Team, Central Science Laboratory, Sand Hutton, York, United Kingdom

Dr Roshini Jayewardene
Office of Chemical Safety, National Industrial Chemicals Notification & Assessment Scheme, Sydney, Australia

Dr Thomas E. McKone
Deputy Department Head, Indoor Environment Department, Lawrence Berkeley National Laboratory, Berkeley, CA, USA

Dr Steve Olin *(Chair)*
Deputy Director, ILSI Research Foundation, Washington, DC, USA

Dr Halûk Özkaynak
Senior Scientist, Environmental Protection Agency, Research Triangle Park, NC, USA

Secretariat

Ms Carolyn Vickers
International Programme on Chemical Safety, World Health Organization, Geneva, Switzerland

Public and peer review

The draft document was published on the WHO/IPCS Internet site for public and peer review comment for three months in early 2007. In addition, a direct mailing campaign to risk assessment institutions and individual experts was undertaken by the Secretariat.

Preparation of final document

The final version of this document was developed in three stages. First, an IPCS Data Quality Review Group considered the public and peer review comments received and prepared a proposed revised document. Second, the additional experts that had been involved in the process of developing the public review draft (see above) were invited to review the document and provide comments. Third, the IPCS Data Quality Review Group agreed on the final document. The IPCS Data Quality Review Group was assisted in its task of finalizing the text by Dr Katherine Walker. Dr Walker's contribution to the project is gratefully acknowledged. The members of the IPCS Data Quality Review Group and those additional experts who provided comments are listed below.

Members of the IPCS Data Quality Review Group

Dr Michael Dellarco
National Institute of Child Health and Human Development, Bethesda, MD, USA

Dr William C. Griffith
Associate Director, Institute for Risk Analysis and Risk Communication, Department of Environmental and Occupational Health Sciences, University of Washington, Seattle, WA, USA

Dr Chris Money
Industrial Hygiene Advisor – Europe, Exxon Mobil Petroleum & Chemical, Machelen, Belgium

Dr Steve Olin *(Chair)*
Deputy Director, ILSI Research Foundation, Washington, DC, USA

Secretariat

Ms Carolyn Vickers
International Programme on Chemical Safety, World Health Organization, Geneva, Switzerland

Dr Katherine Walker
Consultant, Cologny, Switzerland

Reviewers

Dr Nancy B. Beck
Toxicologist/Risk Assessor, Office of Information and Regulatory Affairs, Office of Management and Budget, Executive Office of the President, Washington, DC, USA

Dr Thomas E. McKone
Deputy Department Head, Indoor Environment Department, Lawrence Berkeley National Laboratory, Berkeley, CA, USA

Dr Halûk Özkaynak
Senior Scientist, Environmental Protection Agency, Research Triangle Park, NC, USA

1. INTRODUCTION

The outcomes of exposure assessments are often critical inputs to risk assessments and ultimately to decisions about environmental control of chemicals. Among the questions that must be addressed by an exposure assessment are the following:

- What are the important pathways of exposure?
- What populations or subpopulations have the greatest exposures?
- Should exposure be reduced? Does it exceed some acceptable limit or standard?
- How effective are different alternatives at reducing exposure?
- How uncertain are the exposure estimates necessary to make these determinations, and what are the key sources of uncertainty?

Ensuring the quality of the data in the exposure assessments that are used to answer such questions therefore needs careful planning and examination.

Figure 1 illustrates the role of this document on data quality in the constellation of World Health Organization (WHO)/International Programme on Chemical Safety (IPCS) projects relating to exposure assessment methodology, each of which is highlighted in grey. As the figure suggests, this document is intended as an overarching set of principles relevant to the design, execution and communication of exposure assessments. It should be seen as complementary to the detailed WHO/IPCS guidance on particular elements of exposure assessment also listed in the figure: *Human Exposure Assessment* (IPCS, 2000), *IPCS Risk Assessment Terminology, Part 2: IPCS Glossary of Key Exposure Assessment Terminology* (IPCS, 2004), *Principles of Characterizing and Applying Human Exposure Models* (IPCS, 2005) and Part 1 of this Harmonization Project Document, *Guidance Document on Characterizing and Communicating Uncertainty in Exposure Assessment*.

The figure also acknowledges that the WHO/IPCS guidance documents on exposure assessment methodology are usually components of a larger risk assessment or decision-making context, indicated by the box at the base of the diagram. The needs of the risk assessment or decisions for which exposure assessments are developed are important considerations in defining the data quality requirements for a particular project from the outset. For example, the greater the consequences of a decision, the greater may be the requirements for the quality of the data and the need for communicating to decision-makers the limitations of the data. It might otherwise be acceptable to ignore or discount limitations in data quality in the risk assessment or later decisions that may be based on that risk assessment. The interdependence of these factors is represented by the arrows on either side of the figure.

Four basic hallmarks of data quality—*appropriateness*, *accuracy*, *integrity* and *transparency*—are introduced in this document. These hallmarks of data quality represent basic principles that are applicable in many analytical endeavours but are tailored here to the needs of exposure assessment. Through the introduction of these hallmarks, this document provides a common vocabulary and set of qualitative criteria for use in the design, evaluation and use of exposure assessments to support decisions. This general guidance is intended for use in conjunction with more detailed quantitative methods that exist to establish particular measures of quality (e.g. accuracy and precision, quality assurance/quality control measures).

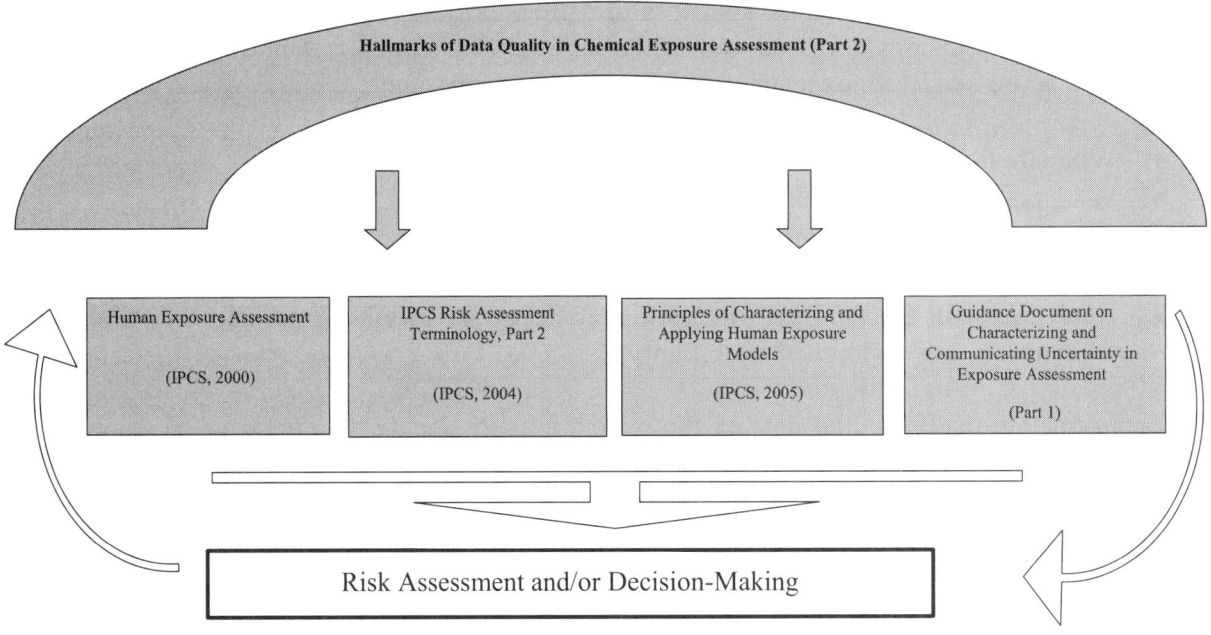

Figure 1: IPCS guidance documents for exposure assessment

Consequently, this document is intended not only for those who carry out the assessments, the exposure assessors, but also for those who incorporate the results into the assessment of risk, the risk assessors, and those who must rely on the final results to make decisions, the risk managers. The introduction of vocabulary and criteria is intended to facilitate communication between these groups or, in the case where one person performs one or more of these roles, to facilitate a more comprehensive thought process. It is hoped that these hallmarks of data quality can be incorporated early on in the development of exposure assessments and can allow risk assessors and risk managers to more quickly and clearly identify aspects of assessments that need more work or further justification.

The remainder of the document is organized as follows. The next two sections lay the foundations for the terminology used in the document: section 2 defines "data" in the context of exposure assessments; and section 3 introduces a broader concept of "data quality" characterized by the four "hallmarks" or measures of quality mentioned above—appropriateness, accuracy, integrity and transparency. Section 4 discusses how these hallmarks might be applied to the design or evaluation of an exposure assessment to ensure its quality. The final section concludes with a broader perspective on the role of data quality in exposure assessment and its importance to risk assessment and risk management decisions.

2. WHAT DO WE MEAN BY "DATA" IN EXPOSURE ASSESSMENT?

For the purposes of this document, the term "data" is defined broadly based on the description of exposure assessment detailed in IPCS (2004) and covers a wide variety of measurements, methods, modelling and survey information relevant to a given exposure assessment. The definition of "data" also includes the many elements of exposure assessment, from the development of *exposure scenarios* to the details of how they are *modelled*, to the selection of model input *parameters* and ultimately to how the results and their uncertainties are characterized and communicated to others (see text box for more detailed definitions).

Definitions of key elements of exposure assessment	
Term	Definition
Exposure scenario	"a combination of facts, assumptions, and inferences that define a discrete situation where potential exposures may occur. These may include the source, the exposed population, the time frame of exposure, microenvironment(s), and activities. Scenarios are often created to aid exposure assessors in estimating exposure" (IPCS, 2004).
Exposure model	"a conceptual or mathematical representation of the exposure process" (IPCS, 2004). The term *model* is used to describe exposure, including all the circumstances, the scenarios and their mathematical expressions.
Parameter	The term *parameter* has several different meanings, ranging from specific to general. In this document, it is used in a broad sense to include physical constants, calibration constants and other inputs to a model that may vary, such as over time, over space or among individuals in an exposed population (see Part 1 of this document).

"Data" are thus considered to be any information that contributes to, or is relevant to, a particular exposure assessment.[3] The term encompasses not just numerical values or estimates, but also information provided in other forms, such as default values adopted for regulatory purposes, theory developed from first principles or basic science, computer programs, surveys, demographic data, census information, graphs, mathematical formulae, subjective expert judgements and descriptive summaries. More detail on the diversity of information that contributes to exposure assessment may be found in the other IPCS risk assessment documents, shown in Figure 1 (IPCS, 2000, 2004, 2005; Part 1 of this document).

We adopt this broad definition to encompass the many and varied approaches often employed in human exposure assessment. Narrower definitions may focus only on measurement data collected in a field or laboratory study. However, such definitions tend to neglect considerations of study design, data processing, analyses and reporting, and the principles, reasons or scientific theories motivating the collection of the values for a given exposure assessment. Adopting this more inclusive definition of data as information, although more challenging, is an attempt both to provide a more global perspective on data quality and to encourage those generating and using exposure assessments to think carefully not just about

---
[3] This definition of "data" is what the United States Office of Management and Budget (2002) Information Quality Guidelines refer to as "information".

individual components of exposure assessment, but about how they work together to create a high-quality assessment.

3. TOWARDS A BROADER DEFINITION OF QUALITY IN EXPOSURE ASSESSMENT: HALLMARKS OF DATA QUALITY

Moving towards a broader definition of "data quality" requires first acknowledging more conventional, but narrower, meanings of the term. To date, formal systems for ensuring and evaluating data quality have primarily addressed specific steps in the process of acquiring, storing and describing numerical data. Many documents on data quality, for example, are focused on a narrower range of questions that deal with judging whether the analysis of samples meets pre-established quantitative criteria for the accuracy and precision of a chemical analysis or other laboratory procedures.

These more specific criteria for data quality are important, but represent only one aspect of the more multidimensional problem of ensuring data quality in exposure assessment. For example, they are not designed to deal with the implications of further use of the data in an exposure assessment or other kinds of assessments. Judgements about the quality of data often depend on the utility of the data for their intended purpose and may change when the same data are used for other purposes. Furthermore, statistical methods can be useful in describing the extent and sources of variability in data, but may not capture major limitations and uncertainties in a data set or the methods used to generate data (see text box for the distinctions between variability and uncertainty). They often assume that other steps in the exposure assessment process are known or can be flawlessly specified. Such characteristics mean that standard data quality systems or statistical methods cannot be relied on as the sole bases for assessing data quality in exposure assessments as it has been more broadly defined in this document.

Distinguishing variability and uncertainty	
Term	Definition
Variability	Heterogeneity of values over time, space or different members of a population, including stochastic variability and controllable variability. Variability is a true or an inherent property of the system or population being evaluated and cannot be reduced by collection of additional information.
Uncertainty	Lack of or "imperfect knowledge concerning the present or future state of an organism, system, or (sub)population under consideration" (IPCS, 2004). May affect its accuracy or relevance. Uncertainty can be reduced, at least in principle, by collecting more information.

In reality, exposure assessors and those who use their results face a range of challenges they must address to evaluate the quality of data chosen throughout the exposure assessment process:

- Is the basic choice of data relevant and appropriate for the specific goals of the exposure assessment?
- Given that they are considered generally appropriate, are the data an accurate measure of the quantity that is being estimated?

- Were the data collected in such a way that their basic integrity has been maintained? That is, have there been errors in the collection, storage and processing of data such that the data no longer represent what they were intended to represent?
- Have the choices and applications of data at each step in the exposure assessment been documented in a clear and transparent manner such that they can be independently understood, evaluated or reproduced by others?

Data that successfully meet the challenges posed in these questions can be said to exhibit certain distinctive characteristics—hallmarks, as we have called them in this document—that are indicative of data quality: *appropriateness, accuracy, integrity* and *transparency*. Table 1 provides a brief overview of the hallmarks, their definitions and some general examples. As the summary table indicates, these four hallmarks of data quality are closely related and may in some cases overlap. In particular, the need for transparency in documentation and communication cuts across each of the other hallmarks. In the paragraphs that follow, we define each hallmark in greater detail and illustrate how implementation of the principles they embody can improve the quality of exposure assessments and the decisions that follow from them.

Table 1: Overview of hallmarks of data quality.

Hallmark	*Definition*	*General examples*
Appropriateness	The degree to which data are relevant and applicable to a particular exposure assessment.	• Exposure patterns (e.g. food intakes, personal activity patterns) that may have been measured in another population, geographic area or other situation are relevant to the current assessment
		• Exposure or dose metrics are relevant to the type of health effects being investigated
		• Exposure models selected or developed are suited for estimating the desired exposure
Accuracy	The degree to which measured, calculated or modelled values correspond to the true values of what they are intended to represent.	• Any sampling programme has been designed to be statistically representative of the geographic area, population, time period, etc.
		• Analytical methods accurately identify and measure the quantity of particular contaminants
		• Any analytical equipment and/or methods and mathematical models used have been calibrated and validated
Integrity	The degree to which the data collected and reported are what they purport to be.	• Quality assurance/quality control programmes are in place
		• In the process of collecting, generating, analysing and reporting data, information is not modified, altered, destroyed or otherwise compromised
		• Samples for chemical analysis are collected, stored and analysed in a scientifically defensible manner
		• Controls have been established to minimize data entry or transfer errors in the development of

Part 2: Hallmarks of Data Quality in Chemical Exposure Assessment

Hallmark	Definition	General examples
		databases
Transparency	The clarity and completeness with which all key data, methods and processes, as well as the underlying assumptions and limitations, are documented and available.	• Study designs, methods, findings and limitations are clearly documented and accessible • Assumptions, equations, parameters, calibration and validation information are documented and accessible • Quality assurance procedures and quality control data are documented and available • Clear rationales are given for interpretations made and conclusions drawn, including rejection of alternative possibilities

3.1 Appropriateness[4]

Whether data or methods used in an exposure assessment can be considered to be of high quality depends, in part, upon the degree to which they are appropriate and relevant to the question at hand.

While this goal may seem self-evident, it may be easily overlooked when an assessment or decision depends on making judgements about hundreds of values and parameters.

Appropriateness of a data set or method is relative to the specific location, scenario, risk assessment or risk management application. For example, data sets collected from a particular geographical region, ethnic group or age group may be of limited usefulness for other regions or groups. Projections of exposure to a chemical released from a particular consumer product, which rely on data on release from a particular matrix of materials under specific conditions or uses, may or may not be relevant to evaluate exposure from the release of that chemical from a different product where these underlying factors are different.

The choice of food consumption patterns to estimate exposure illustrates the role of appropriateness in data selection and evaluation. Methods of analysis or study designs may contain cultural assumptions that limit their usefulness to other cultures. For example, an assessment of dietary exposure to a contaminant in fish may have relied on accurate analytical methods for the contaminant contained in the muscle of the fish and on patterns of fish preparation and consumption typical of a general population. However, these approaches may not be appropriate or representative of exposures for some segments of the population that may consume other parts of the fish, have different methods of preparation of the fish or consume greater quantities of fish compared with the general population. Thus, the same data set might be judged to be highly appropriate for a risk assessment where typical patterns of consumption are the focus, but could be regarded as having limited usefulness in assessing risks to particular population segments.

---

[4] The United States Office of Management and Budget (2002) Information Quality Guidelines include the concept of appropriateness in their term "utility", which they define as "useful and appropriate". We have focused on appropriateness, believing that the data are truly useful only if they are first appropriate and relevant to the question at hand.

A second example is in the choice of an appropriate mathematical method or model. Mathematical methods cover a wide range of techniques, from simple to complex. A simple method might be the use of a dose rate term—for example, milligrams of chemical intake per kilogram of body weight per day of exposure—to represent average annual daily dose. Any variation in daily dose over time is smoothed out by developing the average dose for that period. This metric may be appropriate for health effects for which the average annual daily dose is believed to be determinant of lifetime risk (e.g. some cancers). However, it would not be an appropriate dose measure for estimating a health risk that may depend on the peak or short-term dose (e.g. acute tissue damage).

Evaluation of appropriateness requires a detailed description of the conditions, study designs and methods under which data were collected or information was developed, so that the exposure assessor or other users of the data can judge their relevance for their purposes. An exposure assessor must further document any additional assumptions and simplifications made when using the data in a particular assessment. The determination of appropriateness therefore requires the application of one of the other hallmarks of data quality discussed below, *transparency* (see section 3.4).

Data are most appropriate to use when there is a close match between the needs of the assessment and the characteristics, methods and assumptions underlying the data. Assessment of appropriateness is an important first step towards ensuring *accuracy* of the data, the second of the hallmarks we discuss (see next section). At worst, when data are completely inappropriate, they should not be used. However, in cases when the match is not as close as desired, clear documentation at least allows for an appraisal of the potential bias and/or uncertainty introduced by utilization of the data.

3.2 Accuracy[5]

Accuracy refers to the degree to which measured or calculated values reflect the true values of what they are intended to represent.

Even if data are generally appropriate to a particular assessment, the accuracy of data is ultimately grounded more in scientific and technical factors than in subjective judgements. Technical factors include, among others, sampling design, design of survey instruments, data or sample collection methods, analytical methods, calibration of instruments, validation of models and statistical methods used. The discussion of accuracy in this document is intended simply to draw attention to this aspect of data quality; it cannot supplant the many documents available from national and international organizations on evaluation of the quantitative aspects of the accuracy of data.

---

[5] In the United States Office of Management and Budget (2002) Information Quality Guidelines, accuracy is included in the broader concept of "objectivity", which addresses whether information is " being presented in an accurate, clear, complete, and unbiased manner, and as a matter of substance, is accurate, reliable, and unbiased". The present WHO document discussion of accuracy, however, focuses primarily on the substance—the development and use of data to represent particular exposures. Unbiased presentation of results that are substantively accurate is also critical.

The following examples illustrate some of the steps that occur in the collection of many data sets and the factors that can affect the accuracy of exposure data used to characterize particular exposures.

Given a project with the objective of characterizing the exposure of a population to a given chemical, a first step usually includes design of a statistically valid sampling strategy. Rarely is it possible to measure exposure of every individual in a population, so a subset of individuals must be selected such that the mean and variance of exposure in the subset are an accurate approximation of the mean and variance in the larger population of interest. Such designs can be challenging not only to create, but also to implement in practice. For example, even with the best sampling designs, differential response or participation rates from subsets of the population can lead to unintended biases in the results. Similar issues can arise in the design of sampling programmes to characterize concentrations of contaminants in various environmental media or geographic areas.

Accurate exposure assessments ultimately rely on the accuracy of the methods designed to capture and measure the level of exposure to a contaminant. For example, does a personal monitoring device systematically under- or oversample a contaminant when it is used under field conditions that differ from the laboratory conditions under which it was tested? Have validation data been supplied to allow evaluation of such issues?

Questions about accuracy can also arise from the use of measurement data collected for one purpose that are used for another. For example, investigators and governments often rely on general area sampling of airborne contaminants from fixed monitoring stations in a metropolitan area as a proxy for exposures of individuals. However, numerous factors may affect the accuracy of this assumed relationship (e.g. the locations of the monitors, the mobility of the individuals with respect to the monitors over time, presence of other sources that affect the monitors but not the individuals, exposures of the individual in the workplace or elsewhere that are not picked up by the area monitors).

In all cases, it is necessary that sufficient detail on study design, sampling programmes and implementation be reported with the studies such that their potential influence on the accuracy of the results can be assessed. Exposure assessors are then better able to evaluate and characterize the sources and degree of bias and uncertainty and their influence on exposure assessments.

3.3 Integrity

In essence, the data collected, modelled or otherwise generated and reported are what they purport to be.

Although the integrity of data certainly influences whether they are appropriate and accurate for a particular assessment, it differs from the previous two hallmarks of quality in a fundamental way. An exposure assessment may rely on data that its authors have judged to be generally appropriate and whose methods are accepted as accurate and valid for the purpose for which they were designed. However, if data were not collected, generated, transferred, maintained or analysed in a way that ensures that the expected procedures were followed and that basic information has not been accidentally or intentionally modified, altered or lost, the basic integrity of the data has been compromised. The data, to one degree or another, may no longer represent what they claim to represent.

Maintaining the integrity of data is a primary goal of the quality assurance and quality control policies and procedures used by many companies, universities, and national and international agencies.

Quality assurance policies are generally designed to ensure that the procedures necessary to maintaining the integrity of data are followed. These can vary depending on the application, but may include the development of detailed protocols for each stage of data collection, transport and analysis; the protection of information from unauthorized access to ensure that the information is not compromised through corruption or falsification; the specification of safeguards for the ethical treatment of any animal or human subjects; and the training of instrument operators, survey takers, field data collection technicians and data managers.

Examples of quality assurance protocols that are considered standard practice in any data collection scheme include the use of both internal control samples (e.g. use of field blanks and spikes[6]) and external quality assurance samples (e.g. duplicate samples of known concentrations sent to different laboratories) to determine the extent of intra- and interlaboratory variation. Ensuring that the data have not been compromised or corrupted may also require setting up accessible data archives of original paper or electronic records so that the accuracy of summaries of the data published in documents and articles can be verified.

Quality control procedures are generally established to provide checks on the data that have been collected to evaluate whether in fact the quality assurance procedures were followed and whether the data meet agreed-upon norms. Otherwise, it is difficult for the user to judge the integrity of a data set per se, because there may be few ways to tell that procedures were not followed or values properly recorded. Quality control measures can be linked to the quality assurance procedures. In the example given above for use of field blanks, spikes and duplicate samples, laboratories must provide evidence that their analysis of these samples meets acceptable statistical guidelines for accuracy and precision. Quality control can also simply involve careful analysis of a data set to determine whether it is internally consistent.

As for the other two hallmarks of data quality, integrity of data cannot be assessed or ensured without the presence of the last hallmark of data quality, *transparency*.

---

[6] Field blanks are samples that go through all of the procedures as actual field samples but are designed to have none of the target analyte present, so that if the analyte is found in the blank, contamination may have occurred at some step on the way. Spikes are samples into which known amounts of the target analyte have been introduced; if, upon analysis, the spikes do not exhibit the expected concentrations within statistical norms, the integrity of the field samples may also be in question.

3.4 Transparency

Transparency refers to the clarity and completeness with which all key data, methods and processes, as well as the underlying assumptions and limitations, are documented and presented.

Transparency is an important hallmark of data quality, one that should be represented in every phase of an exposure assessment. Access to key information is necessary not just for the exposure assessor making some initial decision about how to use particular data, but also for the risk assessor or decision-maker faced with evaluating those choices and their implications.

As discussed in the previous sections, transparency is essential for making judgements about the *appropriateness*, *accuracy* and *integrity* of data for use in an exposure assessment. Transparency can help provide the documentation for an analyst to identify and characterize variability and uncertainty. It allows sufficient documentation for risk assessors, decision-makers or stakeholders to reproduce an analysis or conduct sensitivity analyses using alternative data, knowledge or principles as inputs.

Achieving transparency can be challenging. It is difficult to anticipate all the uses to which data might be applied or the perspectives that might be brought to bear on their quality. Consequently, when data are generated or incorporated into assessments, it is essential that a comprehensive description of all inputs, assumptions, processes, models, outputs, limitations, etc., be provided.

Transparent documentation of numerical values may depend on how the numbers were originally generated. Numerical values estimated from a population-based measurement study should describe the study design in detail, the basis for the population sample selected for measurement, how measurements were performed, how values were stored, how statistical summaries of the stored values were calculated, and so on. In other cases, a numerical value in an exposure assessment may be a value that is not associated with any particular data set but has been mandated by regulation or science policy or developed from theory. In this case, transparency requires a description of the source of the value, the types of situations or populations for which it was thought to be relevant and appropriate, any limitations of the value, and the degree and type of uncertainties associated with its use in a particular assessment.

Transparent documentation of assumptions used in exposure assessments is also critical. Most exposure assessments require making a number of assumptions (often made on the basis of reference to other data or situations thought to be sufficiently similar) because of the difficulty and expense of collecting data for all necessary input parameters. Transparency requires that the presence of these assumptions be acknowledged and their rationale and limitations explained. These steps provide the opportunity for the reasonableness of these assumptions to be judged by those reviewing or using the exposure assessment.

The transparency with which data for an exposure assessment have been presented may be judged by answering key questions, such as the following: Would someone who has a general knowledge of the area but is not intimately familiar with the particular methods be able to understand the methods being described? Is the description of the methodology and results complete enough that, in principle, they could be independently replicated or verified by another group? Are the statistical presentations of the data and discussion of assumptions, limitations and uncertainties sufficient that independent sensitivity analyses or characterizations of uncertainty can be conducted?

Ultimately, transparency about the choice of models, methods, assumptions, distributions and parameters is a prerequisite for trust and confidence in the quality of data used in exposure assessments and for credibility of the outcomes of the assessments themselves.

4. FROM EXPOSURE DATA QUALITY TO THE QUALITY OF EXPOSURE ASSESSMENTS

The four hallmarks of data quality in this document were introduced because they are fundamental to the quality of exposure assessments and ultimately to the risk assessments and decisions that depend on them. They represent goals for exposure assessors to strive towards in the development of their assessments as well as important standards for risk assessors and risk managers to use in evaluating the outcomes of the assessments.

Data that exhibit these hallmarks allow their users to answer the basic questions that should be asked of any assessment: Does the choice of data make sense? Is it *appropriate* for the situation? Does it *accurately* describe what it is intended to represent? Is there basic *integrity* in how data are collected and managed sufficient to meet acceptance criteria? Are the presentation and documentation of data *transparent* enough that individuals not involved in generating the data can answer these questions?

All four hallmarks of quality—*appropriateness*, *accuracy*, *integrity* and *transparency*—also reflect factors that can be important contributors to the understanding and characterization of uncertainty in a predicted exposure. What kinds of biases or uncertainties might use of particular data contribute to overall uncertainty? How much uncertainty do they contribute? The quality of data to a large degree determines what approaches, whether qualitative and quantitative, can be taken to characterize uncertainty (see Part 1 of this document).

Hallmarks of data quality are important to the characterization and communication of uncertainty, not just from the perspective of the exposure analyst, but also from the perspective of the target audiences for the exposure assessment. For example, lack of transparency in a source document (e.g. a monitoring study) used in the assessment should be considered by the original investigators as a source of uncertainty, whereas lack of transparency in the report of the exposure assessment may introduce uncertainty or lack of confidence from the perspective of its likely users.

The quality of an assessment—and the degree of uncertainty associated with it—should be evaluated in relation to the decision to be made. Is it sufficient to answer the types of questions with which we began this document? For example, if an assessment predicts exposure to a contaminant to be below the acceptable or other established exposure limit, is the quality of the assessment sufficiently robust to support that finding? Is it possible that the assessment outcome is uncertain enough that the true exposure has a substantial probability of being above the limit?

Part 1 of this IPCS document on uncertainty analysis (section 4.2) suggests a four-tier approach for characterizing the variability and/or uncertainty in the estimated exposure results:

> Lowest-tier analyses are often performed in screening-level regulatory and preliminary research applications. Intermediate-tier analyses are often considered during regulatory evaluations when screening-level analysis either indicates a level of potential concern or is not suited for the case at hand. The highest-tier analyses are often performed in response to regulatory compliance needs or for informing risk

management decisions on suitable alternatives or trade-offs. Typically, higher-tier uncertainty analyses are based on more quantitative and comprehensive modelling of exposures or risks. The highest-tier analyses often provide a more quantitative evaluation of assessment uncertainties that also enables the regulators to determine how soon to act and whether to seek additional information on critical information or data gaps prior to reaching a decision.

In essence, the level of detail and quantification of assessment uncertainties should be related to the quality of the underlying data, the degree of refinement called for in the underlying exposure analysis and decision criteria specified by risk management strategies.

It is important to note that it is not always necessary for all data for, and thus all components of, an exposure assessment to be of uniform quality, as defined by the four hallmarks. Often the magnitude and uncertainty of predicted exposure may be strongly determined by a small number of assessment inputs and be relatively insensitive to others. If it is concluded that the quality of an assessment needs to be improved, it is usually efficient to target efforts towards the data inputs that contribute most to the uncertainty of the output (presuming that uncertainty in this input can be reduced). However, a high level of transparency in discussion of key inputs is always desirable, such that an accurate assessment of uncertainty associated with each input can be made.

The process of evaluating and reporting the quality of information used in an exposure assessment is likely to be an iterative process; as analysts identify and communicate key sources of uncertainties in the assessment results, they may be asked to take steps to incorporate new data and methods, to improve characterizations of variability and/or to reduce uncertainty. Again, however, the need for iterative improvement of an assessment depends on the needs of the decision for which the assessment is designed.

5. CONCLUSIONS

This document contributes to the objectives of the IPCS Harmonization Project by promoting consistency in the quality, presentation and defensibility of exposure assessments used in risk management decisions. It encourages exposure assessors, risk assessors and risk managers to anticipate and to evaluate carefully the quality of data used in all aspects of an exposure assessment.

Four qualitative criteria or hallmarks for judging the quality of data have been described—*appropriateness*, *accuracy*, *integrity* and *transparency*. Attentiveness to each hallmark is critical to the defensibility and credibility of exposure assessments. Thus, exposure assessment should follow the main scientific desiderata of any applied science: empirical testing, data modelling, documentation and reproducibility of results, explicit reporting of assumptions, limitations and uncertainty, peer review and an open debate about underlying theories and models. Transparency is key to the success of all of these steps.

There is a growing appreciation of the need for transparency in exposure assessments as the field becomes more complex. Lack of transparency fails to provide decision-makers with important information relevant to risk characterization and risk management. If, for example, the impact of critical data gaps is not clearly articulated or the degree of conservatism incorporated into an assessment is not clear, the benefits of alternative courses of action may be obscured. Not knowing that an assessment already incorporates several conservative assumptions, for example, a decision-maker might choose to impose additional restrictions on use of a hazardous material without understanding how likely or necessary they are to reduce exposure. With a more transparent accounting of the uncertainties in the data, the decision-maker might choose to assess the potential value of generating additional information to support a more tailored decision rather than make a decision that is constrained by uncertainty. Lack of transparency about data quality can and does result in less than optimum efficiency in allocation of economic and other resources.[7]

Transparency also serves the broader IPCS objectives of international harmonization. Without transparency, comparison among the exposure assessments relied upon by different governments or agencies to regulate a particular chemical or process is difficult. They may rely on particular data, methodologies or assumptions that incorporate different degrees of conservativism and thus lead to different conclusions about risk. Development of common strategies for dealing with hazardous materials or processes, whether as part of environmental programmes or as part of trade agreements, cannot proceed without a common basis of understanding.

Ultimately, the credibility—for scientists, stakeholders and society in general—of the data and assessments on which critical risk management decisions are based owes much to the underlying tenets of data quality discussed in this document. Credibility is a basic element of risk communication and social trust and, in turn, is a determining factor in risk acceptance and risk management.

---

[7] See Part 1 of this document for a complete treatment of this issue.

6. REFERENCES

IPCS (2000) *Human exposure assessment*. Geneva, World Health Organization, International Programme on Chemical Safety (Environmental Health Criteria 214; http://www.inchem.org/documents/ehc/ehc/ehc214.htm).

IPCS (2004) *IPCS risk assessment terminology. Part 2: IPCS glossary of key exposure assessment terminology*. Geneva, World Health Organization, International Programme on Chemical Safety (IPCS Harmonization Project Document No. 1; http://www.who.int/ipcs/methods/harmonization/areas/ipcsterminologyparts1and2.pdf).

IPCS (2005) *Principles of characterizing and applying human exposure models*. Geneva, World Health Organization, International Programme on Chemical Safety (IPCS Harmonization Project Document No. 3; http://whqlibdoc.who.int/publications/2005/9241563117_eng.pdf).

United States Office of Management and Budget (2002) Guidelines for ensuring and maximizing the quality, objectivity, utility, and integrity of information disseminated by federal agencies; notice; republication. *Federal Register*, 67(36): 8452–8460 (http://www.whitehouse.gov/omb/fedreg/reproducible2.pdf).

THE HARMONIZATION PROJECT DOCUMENT SERIES

IPCS risk assessment terminology (No. 1, 2004)

Chemical-specific adjustment factors for interspecies differences and human variability: Guidance document for use of data in dose/concentration–response assessment (No. 2, 2005)

Principles of characterizing and applying human exposure models (No. 3, 2005)

Part 1: IPCS framework for analysing the relevance of a cancer mode of action for humans and case-studies; Part 2: IPCS framework for analysing the relevance of a non-cancer mode of action for humans (No. 4, 2007)

Skin sensitization in chemical risk assessment (No. 5, 2008)

Part 1: Guidance document on characterizing and communicating uncertainty in exposure assessment; Part 2: Hallmarks of data quality in chemical exposure assessment (No. 6, 2008)

To order further copies of monographs in this series, please contact WHO Press, World Health Organization, 1211 Geneva 27, Switzerland (Fax No.: +41 22 791 4857; E-mail: bookorders@who.int). The Harmonization Project Documents are also available on the web at http://www.who.int/ipcs/en/.